IF TEARS COULD SPEAK

WALKING A WIDOW'S PATH

BY

TALLY R. REYNOLDS

Disclaimer

This memoir is based on my personal experiences, memories, and private journals. Some names and identifying details have been changed to protect privacy, but the events themselves remain true to how I lived and recorded them. Conversations and timelines are drawn from both recollection and written notes, and while memory may soften or sharpen some edges, the heart of each story remains as it was.

Everyone mentioned has been made aware of their inclusion, and the thoughts expressed here are mine alone. They reflect how I experienced, understood, and lived through these moments. This book is not meant to speak for anyone else's truth, only my own.

DEDICATION

To those who live on after a love dies.

In memory of my Jack

AUTHOR'S NOTES

If you were curious about this book title, maybe skimmed the back cover, and opened to this page, you may have lost someone with whom you had a beginning, a middle, and then an end. If that is true, let's start there: my sincerest condolences to you, from a heart that knows that emptiness and pain deeply. More than anything else, I want you to know you are not alone in your grief. I am here with mine.

This is not a "How-To" book, unless it is read as "How Did Tally Survive the First Five Years of Widowhood," those horrid, lonely, quiet months without her love, best friend, and husband, Jack. Chapter by chapter, the reader will learn that there was an eventual end to several times an hour weeping, and slowly, so very slowly, whole days were finally lived without a tear. Small things, a song from the past, a mug on a shelf, or a familiar scent, among so many little things, triggered the "us" once created, and I reached for a tissue. A dear friend who lost her husband to a quick, fatal heart attack related how, after almost two years, she cried seeing his spot on a sofa. I said to her, "Oh, I so get that. There will be many moments like that, ones that sneak into what was otherwise a good (or better) day and send you back into grief. I'm sorry. I wish I could tell you otherwise." Her eyes widened. Perhaps she wanted to hear some other words of encouragement. I was a bearer of what would become her "new normal." I knew mine.

From the moment of death to healing, does one ever completely "heal" from this loss, as one certainly never forgets? It is a long path. In these pages, you will see how I walked it, how I found courage, strength, and determination, attributes I didn't know were huddled deep within me until I faced the challenges of being the survivor. I hope for the same discovery for every widowed person.

The widowed might find within these pages our similar experiences from the devastating relationship. I write about what I did with our wedding rings, the clothes in the closet and drawers, vacations, holidays, selling and buying a house, and numerous moments that sent me two steps back in my healing. Did I spark something in fellow survivors of what we have in common, or will one speak to the page, "That's not how I did it?" There are so many ways to get through this loss. Mine is the only one.

The newly widowed, who once stayed up late reading a chapter (or three), may find a diminished ability to remember what happened in the previous pages and give up books of any length. For me, newspaper and magazine articles were barely sufficient; the pile of untouched daily crossword puzzles was eventually tossed into the recycling as I threw up my hands in defeat. Comics were read, but rarely in one sitting. The "Business of Death," as I called the after-the-death piles of paperwork, phone calls, emails, and appointments, sparked grief at every turn and drained one's cognitive abilities. Be patient: reading for enjoyment will return.

Acknowledging the short attention span, all chapters were written as "stand-alone" stories that could be published individually. Later, I melded them into a sequence for this memoir, keeping the redundant details. I know how the widowed brain works, and such a structure allows the reader to read, forget details from the last time reading, and continue, or even skip chapters altogether and start somewhere else.

One of the major struggles as a writer was writing everything in the past tense. Sitting at my desk, the memories came back as if everything had happened today, and words slipped into the present tense. More than once, I was so drawn deeply into the past that, after writing for a while, I stepped out of my new-house office space and was stunned to see its kitchen, expecting the old house with Jack in another room. How my heart and mind wanted everything as it once was. The last chapter is the only chapter in the present tense. It is a letter to Jack from the woman I am now.

There are occasional "F-bombs." Jack's swear words seeped into my daily vocabulary after our retirement from education. A good educator never swore at school, and didn't at home, knowing how easy it would be to carry the profanity to work. Using his F-word brought him back into the room and onto the page, the memories of his frustration with an electrical shock or a bent nail while remodeling, or a chainsaw or his motorcycle that wouldn't turn over. I would be remiss if I deleted them.

I initially attended a group for the widowed offered by a local hospice, a five-week education on what to expect with grief. There was very little sharing of our stories there. Later that first year, I was introduced by a friend to a weekly support group where the widowed spoke of our experiences, which was far more useful; I found I wasn't alone, and it resulted in a lifetime of new friendships. In addition to the support group, I had a skilled therapist to guide my recovery, as well as friends who stood beside me.

My advice is simple: please don't go through the loss alone. Grieving is big, and I mean BIG, on the heart, body, and mind. Reach out. Help is out there, but only when one is ready. Start with a hospice, a church, or a funeral home that may have a support group. I know phone calls are hard to make in the early months. But when you're ready, have had enough alone time, you may want to be with those who know what it is like to lose a loved one.

Know that I care. Walk with me in these pages as you heal and live on.

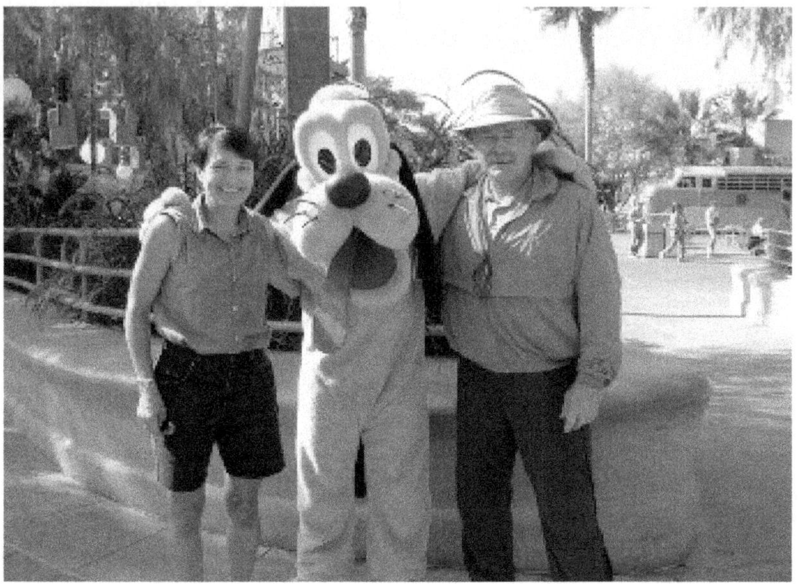

ACKNOWLEDGEMENTS

Before anyone else, I must first acknowledge myself—as egotistical as that may sound—for my own courage to re-enter the dark cave of sorrow and loss and keep writing. I relived Jack's dying and death over and over, page after page. I often stopped writing when the words blurred on the computer screen, when I was in our house, in our bedroom, or at our cabin. My heart felt the hopes of the remissions and then the devastating disappointment when new tumors were found somewhere else in his body. The scabbed hole in my heart was scraped to bleed again. But I wrote and wrote. I earned the accolades that I am a survivor and have lived on.

I have a long list of friends and professionals who encouraged, edited, advised, and impatiently prodded me with, "When are you getting that book done? I want to read it." They pushed me to climb the last mountain to publishing. So here we are.

Two online instructors, names long forgotten, were the springboard for attending in-person classes at two different senior centers near my home. One instructor—another forgotten name, but I can still see her smile and hear her words of encouragement in my mind—saw sparks of a potential writer in me. She knew of a woman in her building, Barbara Haines Howett, who was a published author and an instructor, and contacted her to see if she would take on a student.

Ms. Howett asked for a piece of my writing before our meeting. She, too, saw something in me, and so began six months of honest feedback and, at times, a rough ride as we learned how to dance with my words. I called her "Coach," and she called me "Newbie." We eventually parted ways. I sent her a chapter from the nearly finished manuscript, wanting her approval of how much I had grown as a writer. She emailed back, "You've graduated." Those words still warm my writer's heart. Sadly, she passed away before seeing the completed book she helped start.

My true "graduation" was the result of a single class at Hugo House in Seattle, a memoir class taught by Tara Hardy. Later, she called with an invitation to her private group held for selected memoir writers. "This Tally Reynolds?" I thought, holding the phone. "Are you sure you don't have me mixed up with someone else?" Over many years, chapters were edited by Tara and her group of talented writers who came and went; all gave editing suggestions on chapters submitted to them until the entire manuscript was done. Their honesty and insights truly strengthened my writing, and I learned from the feedback on their submissions to the group, too. Special thanks to those who endured my continuous struggle with verb tenses and still read on.

Again, I want to single out Tara Hardy for her wisdom and talents in helping me become a better writer. It was in her home and on Zoom that those pages formed into this book. Her encouragement when I wanted to quit sustained me through those times of word droughts and "Why bother? Nobody is going to read it anyway" moments.

Referred by Tara, I hired Elena Ellis, who edited the original manuscript. She edited out words that I thought were great ("my roses"), clipped, and trimmed to create a manicured garden.

A special thanks goes to Mary Lou Hill and Maury Hansen, who read the entire manuscript and provided deep insights and suggestions from their own widowed eyes. Hugs to their hearts for the strength and courage to relive their own losses through my story.

Final note of gratitude to the widowed support group in the Seattle-Puget Sound area, WICS (Widowed Information and Consultation Services*). An awkward acronym, but an amazing organization. It provided, free of charge, weekly meetings in the Seattle area—places to share, or just listen when the words were too painful to speak, with others. We learned how much we had in common: the pain, the loneliness, and the silence that overcame us after a death. I wasn't alone in my grief. I met some amazing survivors, some friends for life.

An acknowledgment to Parker Publishers' Tyler Croman, who spearheaded the team of the book cover designer and editors.

*Website for more information: www.kcwics.org

Note: A percentage of the book sale profits will be donated to WICS

To the recently widowed

All the words and sounds in the house are my own now. He took his with him. But I remember his laughter, the warm grasp of his hand on a cool evening walk, the wink of the eye that signaled, "I know what you're thinking." He knew me well.

Learning to live amidst the solitary mental chatter, the tears, and the memories is a difficult lesson. There is no advice from me on how to live on, other than that you will tap a reservoir of courage and strength, previously unknown, and be the survivor you never thought possible in those early days after the death. My way is mine, and so it is with yours.

What I leave is this message for you: keep walking your path. Stumble, fall to your knees in disbelief at what your life has become, run away, and hide, a respite well earned, although I must tell you, grief will find you there.

Keep walking, my friend, just keep walking. Living on will someday become easier.

Contents

Prologue Words:The Day of the Diagnosis.....................................1

Chapter 1 Snapshot: The Last Vacation Memories in a Photo 6

Chapter 2 Still Us: A Moment that Reflected "Us" 13

Chapter 3 Rules: New Rules for Being Uncoupled....................24

Chapter 4 Unspoken: Words Not Said to Each Other 36

Chapter 5 Erasing: The "Business of Death" Burdens.................50

Chapter 6 Envy: Seeing Other Couples 60

Chapter 7 Forgotten: Forgetting A Sacred Date 67

Chapter 8 When: Disposing of His Lasts Meals 74

Chapter 9 Mirror: I Wish I Were a Better Caregiver 81

Chapter 10 Silence: The First Trip Alone....................................90

Chapter 11 The Bed: Memories Around Our Bed......................94

Chapter 12 Poem 101

Chapter 13 Time: Hours and Days Slip Away 104

Chapter 14 One: Selling Our House and His Coffee Mug.......113

Chapter 15 Rings: What Do I Do With Them?.........................124

Chapter 16 Questions: A Cruise Alone and Dating a Passenger
....135

Chapter 17 Later: A New Home and Neighborhood 164

Chapter 18 Poem..184

Chapter 19 Show Up: Therapist and Another Widow's Advice
....185

Chapter 20 Sex and Widowhood: Missing It All.....................211

Chapter 21 Shifts: Third Year and Still Forgetful 218

Chapter 22 Storms: At the Cabin Alone in a Storm 230

Chapter 23 Two: The World is Built for Two............................ 240

Chapter 24 Falling: Skydiving for 60th Birthday Adventure . 249

Chapter 25 Birdhouse: Our Cabin, My Refuge........................ 264

Chapter 26 Swimming: Online Dating Experience 271

Chapter 27 Almost There: Jack's Last Cabin Stay 285

Chapter 28 Poem 295

Chapter 29 Gifts: The Woman in the Mirror 298

Chapter 30 Lessons: What I Learned After Five Years............ 310

Chapter 31 Letter... 327

About The Author.. 338

Prologue
Words: The Day of the Diagnosis

"Tally, Jack's on my line. Says it's important. Pick up when I transfer him over."

The secretary's hand rested on the doorframe as her spectacled face popped in to relay the message. Jack had tried several times earlier to reach me on my personal phone line, she added, before she disappeared back down the hall between the school counselors' rooms and her desk in the main office.

A few seconds later, the call rang in.

I hadn't peeked at the caller ID all day; I only snipped at the receiver with each ring, "You just have to wait your turn." My fellow counselors and I called this "Crazy Friday," referring to the chaos that erupted when every student, staff member, and parent wanted help before the weekend. While I waited for a student, I typed an email to an anxious parent. A loud gurgle from my stomach reminded me that my mid-morning snack and lunch were still in the staff refrigerator, uneaten.

Cradling the phone between my ear and shoulder to free my hands, I ran three sentences together: "Hey, Jackson, what's up? It's Crazy Friday. This has gotta be short." I assumed he was making plans for a dinner date, this was his "important?" so I gave him half my attention while I focused on the computer screen in front of me.

Jack drew out his words. "I'm...at...the...doctor." He sounded far from the phone, in another place. "Remember the mole the doc took off

Monday? The biopsy showed it is..." His voice cracked into sniffles, silence, then heaving breaths.

My hands froze on the keyboard, and the words blurred on the computer screen. I caught the phone receiver as it began to slip off my shoulder. As if a band squeezed around my ribs, I struggled for air. Wild heartbeats clanged a warning: *Get away while you can. Hide.* I wanted to slam the phone down before he could finish the sentence. Why wasn't I somewhere else in the building? I should have gone to the student's classroom to save her the walk to my office. Why did I pick up that damn phone? I wanted to un-hear those words: "The biopsy showed..."

But then the guilt pricked. Why didn't I accompany Jack to the appointment? Why wasn't I with him under the bright fluorescent lights that cast no shadows, when the biopsy results careened off the sterile white walls and shiny chrome medical equipment to pummel my man down to a scared boy? No one should ever hear that news alone. A good wife would have been by his side.

There had been no forewarning that morning, no darkening clouds or silent birds in the yard. We walked through our morning routines as we had done for twenty-three years, clueless, the smell of peanut butter and toast between us. I'd asked him, "A follow-up appointment, no biggie, right?" Jack was a healthy man in his mid-fifties.

"It's nothing," he'd agreed, and shooed me off to work with a kiss. "We'll catch up on news over dinner."

Now, Jack tried to finish the sentence: "The biopsy showed it's...," but his words splintered into sobs.

"Sorry, Bud." My voice grew fainter. "I didn't understand what you said. "

I was truly sorry he had to repeat it. The phone receiver felt pencil-thin in my hand, a numbness climbing from my fingertips into my arm.

He took a long inhale and, on the exhale, said, "…melanoma. Cancer."

A fog filled my office at that moment, dimmed the lights, and hid the stuffed bears, slinky toys, bookshelves, and posters. A chill moved into my mind and body. My lips felt numb. I was a trained counselor, but I had no words of support or comfort for my husband.

"I'm so sorry," fell weakly into the line between us.

I stared out the window at the gray Pacific Northwest day, at the dry blacktop with its white lines for parking spaces, at staff cars of all sizes, models, and colors, at the evergreens and barren maple trees on the other side of the lot. A minivan passed by. Crows scuffled with each other over a brown lunch bag dumped on the sidewalk. The world was normal out there. I wanted to be out there. I wanted everything to stay exactly as it was before I'd said, "Hey, Jackson, what's up?"

My world was organized, neat, and tightly scheduled. I loved the warmth and coziness of our marriage. I enjoyed my staff and students, and the new principal. Jack had the same positive attitude in his role as a middle school teacher in another district. We were each three years from retirement, with sixty-plus teaching years between us. The house was in good shape with new exterior paint and a new roof to keep us dry in Seattle weather, and we had money in savings for the kitchen remodel. Annie B, our Manchester Terrier-Shepherd mutt, was always by our sides; lately, her aging hips slowed our jogs to leisurely walks. All was good.

But I heard Jack say, "Cancer."

Jack said the doctor had scheduled both of us for her first post-lunch appointment at one o'clock.

"I'll be there in thirty minutes," I said to him. "We're in this together."

My eyes flicked to the digital wall clock, with its red numbers and pulsating colon between hours and minutes: 12:23. My school was thirty-five minutes away from the clinic. I was losing time standing there. When did I stand up? My body moved of its own accord, as if it understood I had a new mission: Get to Jack.

I raced from my office. My brown loafers were quiet, cushioned by the industrial-grade blue-gray carpet of the hallway. The main office at the other end suddenly seemed far away. *Please don't let anyone stop me. No crying kids. Don't look anyone in the eye.* At the main desk, I whispered to the other secretary that I was leaving the building immediately.

"Please sign me out. Jack was just diagnosed with melanoma."

Her eyes grew wide. "Oh, Tally, is there anything…"

I did not stay long enough for her to finish. *Run. Get to Jack.*

I had no clue what melanoma was. I felt like a toddler parroting four new syllables: "mel-a-no-ma." Melanoma was the first new word in the avalanche of medical terms and procedures that would threaten to bury us. It was a word that would take over conversations, jolt us awake in the middle of the night, and fill our calendars. It would stealthily hide behind every treatment, pill, and scan, waiting to return.

I did know the word "cancer," of course. Cancer meant something bad was coming. It meant one of us was seriously ill, meant that whatever time remained would be different. As I drove to the clinic, my mind repeated, *Through sickness and in health, and 'til death do you part.* Vows exchanged decades ago, about events I'd always assumed that we would face later, in old age. *Later,* I realized, was *now.*

The drive that December afternoon was the first of many manic rushes to be by Jack's side. My final frenzied drive home would occur on a summer day, four and a half years later, yelling at other drivers with the same impatience and fury.

Get to Jack. In sickness. 'Til death.

Chapter 1
Snapshot: The Last Vacation
Memories in a Photo

Goofy's oversized white gloves rested casually on our shoulders, like we were old pals meeting up in a tavern. His frozen chuckle was stretched wide from one flappy black ear to the other. Hearing, "One, two, three, smile," I squinted at the camera, sunglasses held at my side. Jack's hat cast a soft shadow over his blue-gray eyes. Behind us was a clear aqua sky, filled with shrieks of laughter and fright, the grinding sound of wheels on metal, and a far-off train whistle.

We were celebrating our twenty-fifth wedding anniversary that October in Anaheim. Jack had never been to Disneyland; I had never indulged as an adult. I was born in the area, and my family visited several times. As a child, I savored the pink cotton candy, that sweet smell that pulled onlookers to watch as the food vendor twirled a beehive shape onto a ten-inch paper cone. Would it taste the same forty-two years later? Would the Teacups be as enchanting? I wanted the swish of air tickling my exposed skin, the thrill of g-forces pressing on my chest, and the feeling of being tossed around in the darkness of a tunnel. I wanted to wander in make-believe kingdoms, far away from doctors, treatments, and pills. I wanted Jack to hold me, to feel his warm breath on my ear when he whispered, "I adore you, Talle," at the Happiest Place on Earth.

"Childlike," a colleague once described us. "Not childish," she clarified, "but full of that kid-like spontaneous fun." We were known for our playfulness, like the time we turned off the water of a doomsayer-Y2K-worried neighbor at midnight, or when we instigated an all-out water gun fight with another neighbor after he turned a hose on our passing car. We loved to host neighborhood parties in the cul-de-sac in front of our house, with sidewalk chalk and games for the little ones.

For thirty-six years, Jack had been a middle school teacher, mostly in physical education and health. After seventeen years in physical education, I spent the last fourteen years of my career as a junior high school counselor. Some say you must be nuttier than the adolescents themselves to truly love teaching and coaching this age level, and maybe we were. Thousands of "our kids" passed through our gyms, classrooms, and offices and checked in with us. High schoolers returned to say hello, filled out or slimmed down, some boys showing sprigs of chin hair. Later, some sent Christmas cards, birth announcements, and heartfelt notes, "Dear Ms. Reynolds, I will never forget when you…" It was a rare day when we shopped locally and didn't hear someone yell, "Hey, Mr. Reynolds!"

But it was time for us both to walk away. As our 25th anniversary rolled around, we were both newly retired, just a few months into this new era of our lives.

After shuffling through the airport lines for check-in and security, we bought our ritual airport breakfast of a mocha and a bagel and read the morning paper until the call for boarding.

On the plane, Jack plopped into the window seat, and I took the middle. I prefer the window, too. I love the rush of flying through clouds into sunlight, watching the shadow of the plane streak over string-like rivers and highways. But when he offered to switch seats, I insisted, "No, you take it. I'm going to read my book." Days loomed ahead when I would make reservations for one. On this trip, I wanted the best for him. We squeezed hands and exchanged quick kisses as the plane ascended.

Our hotel was only a hundred yards from the park. Upon arrival, we changed out of flying clothes and walked immediately to the entrance with our three-day passes in hand.

We strolled down various streets. At every junction, in every shop and line, simple musical tunes filtered through crowd noise. Notes of flutes, pipe organs, tubas, and trumpets floated around us like butterflies. I was disappointed that the Ferris wheel, roller coaster, and Magic Mountain were under repair, but I heard Jack's sighs of relief. Unlike me, he never enjoyed racing through curves or anticipating sudden drops from great heights.

When we came across Goofy, a Japanese family was setting up their shot. The parents corralled two toddlers onto Goofy's knees, cooing as the children's wide eyes edged toward panic. The father knelt with a sophisticated camera pressed to his eye. The mother spoke to her children in Japanese, and I guessed from her tone that she was pleading for smiles. I wanted to help, so I made faces and hopped up and down behind her in attempts to pull giggles out of the children. After several clicks from the father's camera, both children raced away from Goofy to their mother, clinging to her legs.

Something came over me, an intuition, and I asked Goofy to stay. I asked the father to take our picture, handing him our palm-sized camera.

Jack was the younger of two children, the only son, and great at posing for photos. I was one of six children; given the cost of film development, my family photos typically included as many siblings as possible. When it came to Jack and me, besides wedding pictures, there were only a few photos of both of us, because I usually operated the camera. Already today, we had passed up the chance for photos with Sleeping Beauty, Mr. and Mrs. Mouse, and a few pirates. But now here we were with Goofy, the perfect character for dog lovers. Without our dog, Annie B, Goofy was our stand-in, the closest we could come to a family shot.

Next to Goofy, I was dressed in black jean shorts and a faded purple sleeveless top, with tan lines already forming. Jack usually burned while I tanned. On this day, he wore a long-sleeved sky-blue windbreaker, navy-colored pants, and a wide-brimmed tan hat, an expensive outfit made of a material that protected him from ultraviolet rays. We played in the sun a little longer than usual that week at Disneyland, as if his outfit had the power to prevent new melanoma tumors.

As if.

At the time of the trip, we were eight months into yet another remission. The fear of relapse was always in the shadows. If the cancer returned, how many more treatments or surgeries could Jack's body take? The collapsing veins of his arm, they used only one, because all the lymph nodes were taken out of the armpit of the other, needed a reprieve from blood draws and chemo. We needed a reprieve from calendars and clocks set around doctors, labs, and treatments.

Near the line for Splash Mountain, the high-pitched squeals of children rained down on us. As the cars careened into standing water, small rainbows flickered in falling droplets while the riders became drenched. We had scheduled this ride for the midday sun, anticipating that we would get wet.

"Sounds like the kids are having fun," I laughed, missing the energy and rambunctiousness of junior highers. How contagious their laughter was.

"Unlike that little shit over there," Jack lifted his chin in the direction of a five-year-old boy wailing at a trinket stand.

"I want that! I want that!" The child's feet stomped fury into the pavement, and his hands flapped the air. A woman pacified him with a sword from a barrel.

"Just wait until he sees a Buzz Lightyear or a cowboy hat," I muttered.

Jack smiled in agreement and whispered in my ear, "I wouldn't want that kid in my class."

"And I wouldn't want that parent on my caseload."

"Not our problem anymore, is it?" Jack shrugged his shoulders, head tilted to one side.

No more time for those kinds of problems, I thought.

Most of the lines moved quickly, allowing us to repeat our favorites: The California Adventure and Indiana Jones. Jack paled when I wanted to do the Haunted Mansion, a ride in which the elevator swoops down floors and opens to something that makes everyone in the entire car scream.

"Chicken," I teased.

"I don't mind them feathers," he retorted, plopping onto a bench in the shade and waving me back into line.

I glanced back: with his legs stretched out and sipping water, Jack was already people-watching. I worried about tiring him out while I felt energized. I wondered if I should stay behind, but Jack would think he was ruining my fun. So I just got on the ride.

By our third day at the park, most of the rides had lost their novelty. Sitting in our room with a sub sandwich and iced tea, out of the midday sun, we did our end-of-trip ritual: a round of "The Bests."

"Which was the best ride?" California Adventure.

"Best breakfast?" IHOP's pancakes.

Best lunch, best dinner, best laugh, most ridiculous tourist.

We rested in anticipation of evening fireworks. As the tourists filled Main Street in front of the trademark castle, Jack slipped his arm over my shoulders, pulled me tight against him, and kissed the top of my head. I nestled my head into his chest and listened to his strong heart. Shifting to be side by side, I wrapped my arm around his back and hooked my thumb on the waist of his denims. A regular guy wearing ordinary jeans, no reminder of the sun-protective clothing already packed for tomorrow's early flight home. Our "oohs" and "aahs" blended with other spectators as the explosion of colors and sparkles cascaded from the sky.

Later that night, under the soft blue glow of a digital clock, I watched his barrel chest rise and fall while he slept. I imagined scenarios like today, but without him. Tears raced down my face as I prayed, *"Please, God, more time."*

One month was all we got after Disneyland. On the Monday after Thanksgiving, a CT scan shattered the hope for a long remission;

cancer was on the move again. My life's worst ride was ahead, without an option to get out of line.

Chapter 2
Still Us: A Moment that Reflected "Us"

The fluid in Jack's abdomen restricted him from getting up or turning over in bed, a side effect of late-stage melanoma. A medical procedure held a sprig of hope in restoring temporary comfort: a long needle inserted into his midsection to draw out what we jokingly called "Buddha Belly." Although the bloating would return in a few days, those few days were gifts desperately needed. The appointment was in two hours, and I needed every second to get Jack up and dressed and to drive the twenty-five-minute route to the doctor's office at a Seattle medical clinic.

When Jack winced, I winced too, as if my own intestines were compressed and twisted along with my husband's. In my fight with God, listening to Jack's moans, I murmured, "Hasn't he had enough?" What could I do to rescue a drowning man from the fluid pooling within him? Like bailing out a boat with a huge hole, far from shore, there were two options: sink, or fill one bucket at a time and toss the water overboard for as long as it takes.

I leaned over Jack's still body in our bed, rubbed his shoulder, and greeted him with the newest of his nicknames: "Time to get up, Buddha Man."

He grunted, and his eyes remained shut.

"You have a doctor's appointment. You gotta get up."

Pain radiated from Jack and pricked the hair on my arm. I had the cruel task of getting him on his feet when all his body wanted was sleep.

His eyes opened slightly, into blue-gray slits. He dragged a heavy hand out from under the teal-colored flannel sheet, and with his palm, he rubbed a small circle around his protruding stomach. "Bud…dha…Bel…ly," he whispered, then slowly smiled and closed his eyes.

Damn it, God!

I wanted to race from the house, throwing fists and shouting at the clouds. Or hurl something fragile against a wall just to hear the shattering. I wanted to roll up in a ball, hold my aching heart, and cry. I felt stabbed with guilt as well as grief. I needed respite from his cries of discomfort. Was this appointment really for Jack, or me?

I pulled the sheets down and kissed his bald head. "Now, Jackson. Now, Bud. Time to get going."

With Jack's diminishing mobility, getting him out of bed had become a slow, elaborate process:

Step 1: With Jack lying on his side, move his feet to hang over the bedframe.

Step 2: Link my elbow to one of his and pull him up sideways to sit with his feet on the floor.

Step 3: Rest.

Step 4: Interlock our elbows and pull him onto his feet.

Step 5: Rest.

Step 6: Walk together, ten feet to the bathroom, my hand cupping his bony forearm and elbow, the other hand grasping the skinfolds at his waistline.

Step 7: Rest on the toilet.

Step 8: Lock arms again to get him to his feet.

Step 9: Rest.

Step 10: Back to bed.

Those rare times he needed to go to the main floor, the fourteen stairs took us several minutes, a grunt with each step. "In sickness. And in health." Seeing Jack so helpless, my once robust and active husband, unable to get out of bed without my assistance, sent out a drumbeat warning inside my chest. He was slipping away. When did this new routine begin? Two weeks ago? A month? I couldn't remember. The small losses accumulated, like autumn falling leaves, until one day the barren tree became the new normal.

What would the next "new normal" be? Images of a totally bedridden man flickered before me: diapers, a bedpan to empty, wipes after a bowel movement, bedsores if I neglected to rotate him frequently. Would hospice provide me with instructions? I only knew what I had seen on the television hospital series. I racked my brain to remember comments from friends with older parents in nursing homes. I had enough financial resources to bring in weekly help, but not enough for residential nursing care. Our plan was to sell the house and use the profits for his long-term care, since he did not qualify for the plan that my school district offered employees and spouses. His diagnosis came one week too soon, and he was denied enrollment. The idea of moving sent chaos swirling in my mind: packing alone, selling the house, and finding an apartment for myself.

No future tripping. Get him to the doctor.

Jack was notably worse this morning. I had to work harder to get him out of bed and onto his feet. As we descended the staircase to the garage, I muffled my grunts and managed a perky, "Almost there."

Jack groaned, "Slow down," then snapped, "Stop. I need a rest."

When we arrived at the medical building, we navigated another first: Jack was unable to walk from the parking spot to the doctor's office. I dropped him off at an entry bench, parked the car, and then ran into the lobby for a wheelchair.

A wheelchair? I wanted to beg, try harder, and walk the hallway with me. It's not that far. I wanted my healthy man back. Instead, I easily lifted Jack's feet onto the footrests. I was stunned by how lightweight his legs were, hidden under his sweatpants. Until that moment, I had no idea how much of Jack was already gone.

We traveled the long hallway to the elevators, with framed pictures of painted flowers against the washed-out yellow walls, a decorator's attempt to bring nature into a windowless corridor. Pine-scented disinfectant masked the scent of the sick, injured, unwashed, and scared. Typically, this hall was busy with medical personnel and patients, but today we were greeted by an eerie silence. Only the soft hum of rubber wheels along the gray linoleum announced we were here. Jack sagged into the cracked vinyl seat. Instead of his hand, which I'd held en route to every previous appointment, I held the cold handles of the chair.

His hands gripped the arms of the wheelchair. These were the same hands that had remodeled our homes, added windows and walls, and made my designs a physical reality. These were the strong hands that once soothed and caressed me. But this morning, these hands were fumbling with shirt buttons, unable to get dressed without my help: shirt, socks, shoes, pants. I flashed on Jack's weary eyes as I tied his shoes and saw, *I'm sorry you must do this.*

I pushed his wheelchair, looking at the back of his head in his Boston Red Sox baseball cap. He wasn't a Boston follower, but he delighted in how it irked local Seattle-area Yankee fans. The stubble of hair underneath had only begun to come back a month ago, after his last radiation treatment, the final attempt to stop the growing tumors now settled in his brain. Was it the chemicals from the treatment that made it all silver, with no trace of the reddish-blond it once was? If he had been healthy, what would his natural color be today? Although we were only four years apart, we often snickered that my salon brunette coloring job made it appear that Jack had hustled and married a much younger woman. *Won't we be a cute silver-haired couple in our seventies, when I let my hair go natural?*

His Cannon Beach fleece jacket did little to hide the skin sagging around his neck, the drooping shoulders, or sleeves filled with more air than muscle. I had a matching jacket, our second set of matching coats. Early in our courtship, he bought us pullover windbreakers. I panicked: *How serious is this relationship to wear matching jackets in the second month?* My jacket was the wrong size, but the relationship fit. It was only six months from the first date to the wedding day. Now our twenty-seventh wedding anniversary was only a few months away. This year, there would be no dinner out, no romantic walk along the waterfront, no hand-delivered flowers.

We rolled past the dark conference room in the hall. On the door was a printed sign: "Leukemia Support Group at 10 a.m." Was there a "Melanoma Support Group?" Would I be sitting in a fluorescent-lit room at a table with other caregivers someday, telling my story about how much I loved this man and how I missed him so deeply?

No future tripping. Stay here with Jack.

What was he thinking about, being unable to walk the short distance to the doctor's office after being such an athletic man? What a defeat for those muscular legs that had played high school football, wrestled, taught physical education, and carried him on our nightly jogs and walks. Now he needed a wheelchair. How could he rationalize what was happening to his body? God knows I couldn't. But Jack clutched his thoughts deep inside on that ride, locked in and locking me out.

In the four years since his diagnosis, Jack had refused any conversation about dying and death, as if talking about it would dent the armor he'd worn against his mortality.

When the CAT scan revealed more tumors, we faced the fact that all available treatments had failed. Jack would eventually die from this cancer.

"So, what are you thinking?" I inquired hours after we'd received the news. My heart pounded in my chest. I knew that I was risking a confrontation with him, but thought perhaps he would talk to me this time. *Please talk to me. I don't want to do this alone.*

Silence. Jack stopped in the hallway, statue-like.

"Talk to me, Jack. This is the beginning of the end." I placed a soft hand on his back, but feeling the cold that radiated from him, I pulled back.

Silence.

God, give me the words so I can get him to open up to me. This ain't working.

I stepped in front of him, softening my voice to just above a whisper. I jumped to Counseling 101 and focused on my own feelings. "Are you scared? I know I am."

"Damn right I am! I shouldn't be dying." Spit flew from his lips, hitting my chest. I wiped it away as Jack turned from me, heading to the basement to hide in some television show.

"Everyone has to go sometime, Babe. You just get to know how."

Jack stomped back toward me, a hard glare into my eyes. "Well, not me!"

My weariness took over. I waved my hands into the air and spewed, "What makes you so special that you won't die like the rest of us? Welcome to the human race!"

Oh my God, what did I just say? I struck a dying man. Wrong, wrong, wrong, Tally. Say something. Apologize.

His face flushed, lips pressed into a line, eyes glaring. He about-faced and stormed down to the basement. I went into the kitchen, sat on the new barstools, and tried to figure out what had gone wrong.

He said nothing more about dying. Ever.

Maybe it was too much for Jack to see all the sorrows and joys of a lifetime end, those adventures for another day, a later time that would never come. Maybe he was protecting who he thought he was to me, the man, the protector of his woman. I wish those defenses could be drained along with the abdominal fluid. I needed to hear his heart speak. We needed to talk freely.

Obviously, I wasn't very good at starting or guiding the conversation. With several tumors in his brain, there was the possibility of a stroke, leaving him speechless or dead. Neither of us wanted angry words in what time was left. So I stayed silent too. But the words I had to say hummed like a hive in my head:

What were your fondest memories?

Any regrets?

What shall I do with your ashes?

Any favorite songs for the Celebration of Life?

Anything special of yours I should give to your sons?

Please tell me you adore me. Again and again.

Walking up the clinic corridor, I remembered that only six weeks earlier, we had been on the East Coast for Jack's sixtieth birthday, a surprise trip.

Early in our marriage, Jack proved unable to take hints about birthday gifts, even when I resorted to circling items in ads to indicate gifts I might like to receive. After receiving ill-fitting or ugly clothing, tools I didn't need, and trinket-like jewelry, I came up with a new strategy: surprise adventures. The birthday celebrant would never know what was up until the arrival at the destination. We gifted each other biplane rides, dinner trains, whale-watching boat trips, and a Russian submarine tour, and dozens more. Creating a memory together was better than any wrapped item.

Jack knew nothing of our last trip, only what to pack. I handed him the itinerary for the week when we landed in Chicago, en route to New York and Washington, D.C. He sounded like a child at Disneyland, bubbling over with "Wow!" and "Oh, you gotta be kidding me!" We spent time in taxis and on a hop-on, hop-off bus, and took short strolls through Broadway, Little Italy, Arlington Cemetery, the Smithsonian, and the Korean and Vietnam memorials.

I watched him search for a high school classmate who died in Vietnam, a war Jack missed by a few draft numbers. Jack's plan, if drafted, was to run to Canada, unlike his father and grandfather, who served in the World Wars. He carried embarrassment decades later, thinking himself a coward to entertain the idea of running from duty, a near miss at disgracing the family name. Yet he was self-aware enough to know that he could not kill another being. I loved his soul, the compassion it held for life and the living.

It had only been six weeks, six weeks from a hop-on, hop-off bus to a wheelchair. Too fast. He was dying too fast.

We passed several windowless doors along the medical center hallway: "Staff Only," "Supplies," and "Custodial." As I pushed, I realized this was the first of what would be many more wheelchair rides. Where do I rent one? How will I get it into and out of the car by myself? How does one get a handicapped parking permit for a car? I imagined the eventual hospital bed, the commode in the house, and moving him from the upstairs bedroom to the main floor living room.

Despite my organization, planning, and anticipation of his needs, I could not control the inevitable. I was reeling from the constant changes. As soon as I had his pills organized into morning and evening pill containers, and a spreadsheet with check-off boxes, a medication was dropped, and a new one added. "Four times a day," "twice a day," "morning and night," "with meals." And the bottle that simply stayed out all the time: "For pain as needed." Then came the morphine pills, the last option for pain management. That bottle's label had an invisible warning: The final days are nearing.

I was a mere leaf, aloft for as long as the wind blew.

The chair weaved like a grocery cart with one bad wheel. My five-foot-five-inch frame clumsily steered Jack's five-foot-ten-inch frame into corners and walls, causing him to flinch and cry out. I wished he would throw his hands up, rise from the chair, and yell, *Jesus Christ, let me steer. You're going to kill me before we get there!* And we would laugh and laugh. I wanted to laugh.

Heading straight into the elevator, the space was too small to turn the chair around. Our backs were to the closing doors. We were quiet on our ride up to the third floor. This was the same quiet I'd been living with these last two months, with Jack sleeping most of the day. The basement, where Jack typically watched TV, went unused. The long kitchen counter, designed to allow us to easily work side by side during meal prep, was used only for placing items pulled from the refrigerator or microwave. There were no cookies baking, no huge salads, no aromas of marinara sauce and garlic bread for Italian dinners.

So, this is what it will be like after he is gone, I kept thinking, listening to the silence. The chores, the house maintenance, and the dog care will all be mine. There will be no one to tease, make plans with, or touch. The car rides will be quieter, too, without our silly language about seeing dogs outdoors in yards, all noted in military terms: "Sentry" meant a dog was sitting on the front door stoop, also nicknamed "Duty Dog;" "Recon" was a dog who walked along a fence or yard. Dogs playing in the yard were on "R&R." Passing nursing calves, Jack would say, "Someone is getting juice." My vocabulary had become augmented with Jack's funny way of phonetically saying words: "fat-a-cue" (fatigue), "ass-per-gus" (asparagus), "phee-no-meal" (phenomenal), and others. Chuckling, Jack would praise me, "I'm so glad you're saying it right."

But now it was quiet. Painfully quiet.

I pulled myself back from the past and the future into the elevator, only to find my hands white-knuckled, holding onto the chair. I was just holding on. Tears began to gather, and I fought them back. I wanted to be strong for him, wanted him to believe that I, too, believed he had more time.

Right here, right now. Our mantra began its rhythmic drumming because he was still here, my Jack, too weak to walk, but here.

Stay out of the future.

With a familiar chime, the elevator doors opened on the third floor. As I began to pull the chair out backward, it was as if a choir director's baton had pointed at both of us. A duet of "doot-doot-doot," the sounds of a commercial truck in reverse gear, sprang simultaneously from our lips, followed by our laughter. We'd thought the same thing at the same time.

Regardless of all the cancer had thrown at us, we were still us.

Chapter 3
Rules: New Rules for Being Uncoupled

If I had known Jack's last breath and heartbeat were five hours away, I would have never left the house.

A large rotating fan hummed in our lofted bedroom that morning. We were in the midst of an early summer heat wave, and warm air swirled around Jack. Before leaving for soccer practice, my team was preparing for a national tournament, I covered the tall windows with newsprint, adhered with painter's blue tape. Uncovered, the southern exposure windows baked the house from one in the afternoon until the sun slid behind the greenbelt, tall cedars, and evergreens in the early evening. Guilt passed through me. Getting new blinds that could open and shut by remote from the ground floor was on my "to-do" list. What minor tasks had kept me from calling the window blinds company? Pulling weeds? Wiping food splatters from the microwave? Finishing a Sudoku puzzle?

From the top of the ladder, over the low wall of the lofted bedroom, I saw Jack on his side, facing away from me on the bed. The pale skin of his exposed right shoulder and upper back contrasted with the teal flannel sheet bunched around his waist. I chatted over the wall between us.

"It's getting warm already, isn't it?"

A weak, "Yeah," drifted up from the bed. Jack did not turn to face me.

"Kim is coming over today to watch you while I'm at practice. Is that okay?" Kim hadn't seen Jack for years, and I worried she might not be ready for what cancer and treatment had done to her former colleague: the weight loss, no hair on his head. Maybe his vanity wouldn't want her to see him like this.

There was a long pause, and then another soft, "Yeah."

"I'll be gone for only two hours. Don't decide to go out for ice cream without me, okay?"

This time, "Yeah" came with a burp-like chuckle.

"Want any Jell-O before I go?" I knew the body wanted only water at the end.

Please, God, make him want something.

"Nah."

I wanted to nag him until he gave in to eating a little. Change your mind, please. Want something. In the final month, Jack's needs had become simplified: long naps, toast, and mashed potatoes evolved to Jell-O, Gatorade, and iced tea, until it was only sleep, ice chips, and morphine.

"Sure?"

"Yeah."

He was still cognitively with me then. There was still time for me to leave him.

I clung to the Hollywood script of the dying husband's last moments:

WIFE kneels at the bedside, holding HUSBAND'S hand in hers. They share a final kiss and look longingly at one another. WIFE bends down to hear a whisper from his dry lips.

HUSBAND: I adore you.

WIFE: I love you so much, and places her other hand on the side of his face.

The camera draws in on the husband, slowly closing his eyes. As his body relaxes, he gives one final exhale. She watches the pulse at his neck until it stops.

WIFE: (tears fall as she lays her head on his chest.)

Anything contrary to this movie ending was walled off by my denial. I was the good wife who didn't want to face the alternative, struggles for breath, pain spasms, or final pleas for relief. I was frightened at how helpless I was, powerless to alleviate his discomfort. All I could do was watch and cry and pray until the end. I held onto the Hollywood death fantasy until it was almost too late.

Other than the movie in my mind, my father's death was all I knew. Like Jack, cancer took Dad in his young sixties. Dad's cancer was self-induced lung cancer from decades of tobacco use, while Jack's skin cancer was triggered by years of sunburn on his fair skin. But their stories ended differently. Dad became comatose two days before his end, while Jack walked to the bathroom on his last night, albeit slowly and painfully, with my help. On Dad's final evening in the hospital, his kidneys ceased to operate, as thousands of dead cells became trapped in the body and leaked a stench through his pores. A nurse informed us that his body was shutting down; his death was near. I didn't have those warnings with Jack at home. I assumed there must be more time.

The visiting hospice nurses gave me no information about how life leaves the body. But I didn't ask or research either. I didn't want to know. I wanted to believe, each morning, if Jack is still here with me now, surely he will still be with me tonight. Day after day. I wanted to believe the oncologist, who said three months ago, "Maybe another year." I wanted to believe the hospice nurse who ventured last week that Jack should have another month or two. I wanted to believe her yesterday's "Another week, maybe two." I wasn't ready. Not this weekend.

Fifteen minutes from the house, five minutes from the practice field, my cell phone rang. Kim's breath was short and hard, as if she were sprinting. Her panic became mine: "I think you should get back here now. I think it's close."

Swearing at red lights, swearing at slow drivers, swearing at walkers in crosswalks, I made it to the park, threw soccer gear to a teammate, and yelled, "I gotta go!" and raced home.

I took the stairs two at a time to the bedroom.

"See his leg?" Kim pointed out.

I gasped. That morning, I had tried to put Jack's leg, hanging over the bedframe, back onto the mattress, but was stopped by his pained cry. It was the same leg I bumped into twice earlier that morning, attempting to give Jack sips of water, a few ice chips. Both times, he groaned, and I apologized. I saw the leg as something that should go back under the covers, that should be hidden away with the rest of his ailing body. I did not look at it for signs of dying.

"My grandmother just died last week. They call it 'marbleizing.'"

If I had known to look for the watercolor swirls of pinks, reds, and blues from the blood pooling in his extremities, I would have never left him that day. Ignorance is not bliss; it's just the thin coat of ice over Hell, waiting for a step, a crack, and the fall into brutal reality.

Jack was still lying on his left side, his left arm beneath his head, his right shoulder bared. I left him that way before leaving for soccer. He hadn't gotten up to go to the bathroom since last night. He was becoming still.

Before I left for practice, Jack resisted his morphine pill, spitting it out as I laid it on his tongue, holding the cup of water with a straw for a sip. "Please take it, Jack," I whispered. "It will help with the pain." But again, he slipped the pill off his tongue with his front teeth, letting it fall to the pillow. Was he pain-free and didn't need it? Did it taste terrible?

"Talk to me, Jack, tell me what to do."

But he was becoming quieter.

Standing with Kim, I felt my face flush, my words stuck on my tongue. I, Jack's wife, a good wife, had left his side. I had almost missed his death. I was angry that I didn't know the signs of death. Who was supposed to tell me these things?

Shortly after I returned, the hospice nurse stopped in again, less than eighteen hours from her last visit. She administered a morphine pill anally and sent Kim to the pharmacy to get the liquid version. As I escorted the nurse out, she stopped at the doorway, put her hand on my arm, and gazed directly into my eyes.

From a faraway place in my mind, I heard the nurse say, "It might be this weekend, maybe Monday, Tally." My sense of control dissolved.

No, no, no.

The doorbell rang. Pulling tears back, I opened the door to see my stepson, Steve, and his wife, Kelly. Where were the people selling magazine subscriptions or religion when you needed them? People you could shut the door on. I wanted to close out the world.

Steve stooped to give me a hug. He had Jack's wide shoulders and barrel chest, the same blue-gray eyes, the same red-blonde hair color, when he wasn't shaving his head to hide hints of early balding. Steve was taller than Jack and clean-shaven, unlike his father, who always wore a trimmed mustache. I saw Jack in his thirties when I looked at Steve.

Our relationship had always been friendly, no Mother's Day cards or birthday gifts, but cordial and polite. I was the one who nudged Jack to drop in to see Steve at work, urging him to make time to chat with his son. Jack's cancer diagnosis layered my reminders with urgency, as both men made the effort to see each other regularly.

Today was meant to be a drop-in visit. Steve, too, thought he had more time with Jack. What words could a stepmother offer to a man who came for a quick hello and instead would watch his father die?

While I relayed the nurse's information to Steve and Kelly in the entryway, I heard what I thought was Jack coughing. Then, as if being pricked, I knew what it was: his death rattle. Jack had waited for me to leave the room to slip away, trying to save me from the final moments, his last act of love. But the three of us rushed to the bedside to witness his last breath and heartbeat.

I leaned into Jack. "Tried to sneak off on me, huh? I'm here."

Steve, Kelly, and I each told him he could go.

"I will always love you." I kissed his head.

"I love you, Dad," Steve said. Kelly mumbled words through her sobbing.

The hospice nurse had left a phone number the day before, instructing me to call "immediately upon death." Her voice sounded as if she was speaking from far off in the woods, her words floating up like vapor. I heard the word "*death*" as if we were talking about a winter storm in the middle of June, something to happen much later, something that wasn't about Jack. I put the paper on an ever-growing pile of items to be dealt with eventually.

With what I thought was Jack's last breath, I raced downstairs to the kitchen phone. I wanted to save Steve from hearing the details of the call from there in the bedroom. I assumed the urgency of the instruction, "call immediately," had something to do with the coroner's procedures, an accurate time of death on the certificate, and evidence proving I hadn't rushed the death. My tongue and lips felt Novocain-numb as I mumbled, "He has died, he has died."

Oh, my God. "He has died," I repeated, louder.

"I'm sorry," responded the woman on the other end of the line, terse, desensitized from answering too many of these calls.

"You have twenty-four hours to have the remains picked up."

My hand tightly squeezed the phone. "Remains?"

Remains was what they called him. Not Jack or Mr. Reynolds. Not even *your husband.* He wasn't a person anymore, but remains, like a forgotten coat or a missing cell phone left behind at a restaurant, an item that would remain in the lost and found until picked up.

I yelled back, "He has not been dead for five minutes. Can I have a little time with him?"

"Yes, you can. But you have twenty-four hours to have the remains picked up." Her voice was clipped. Damn her. Damn them all.

I grasped the phone in my hand like I was holding a gardening tool or a hammer, standing anywhere other than the kitchen. I placed the receiver back in place. Twenty-four hours to say goodbye.

From upstairs came Steve's voice, urgent and scared, a grown man losing his father.

"Tally, Tally! He's still breathing."

I dashed up the fourteen stairs, but by the time I was back by Jack's side, there were no more breaths. It was over. Kelly, with her hand on Steve's shoulder, cried for all of us. Steve and I were tearless, blankly staring.

Sitting on the bed, I kissed Jack's head. "Bye, Jackson."

Steve said, "I love you, Dad."

Regret was sharp; I had left the bedroom before I was sure Jack had passed. I put the rules, that instruction to "call immediately," ahead of my presence at my husband's final earthly moments. What kind of wife was I?

Years before, at the open-casket funeral for Jack's mother, I left a goodbye kiss on her forehead. Her waxen body returned my affection with a chill I couldn't forget. I knew I needed to hold Jack one more time while he was still warm. I didn't know how much time I had before he would become cool to the touch. I didn't want a memory of my warmth against his coolness.

After Jack's last heartbeat, I slid into bed behind his body. Jack and I hadn't slept together for days because he'd needed the space to rock, roll, toss, and turn himself into some impossibly comfortable position. I needed one more time together with him. My chest pressed against his back, spoon-style, taking this familiar position for the final time. With my arm draped over his shoulder, I placed my palm on his chest. I felt him cooling. I will miss caressing these hairs, feeling them against my back before falling asleep. Shock dammed sorrow from my eyes. Thoughts were dammed, too. The only words that came were the same words I always said whenever I left the house, every night before sleep came.

I whispered into the silence, "I will always love you."

Early afternoon sun filtered through the maple and evergreen trees out back, creating a mosaic pattern on the maroon cloth blinds above the headboard. I watched an occasional wisp of wind shift the design like a kaleidoscope. The outside, so alive with light, color, and movement. Death inside.

I didn't stay long in bed; too eerie, no matter how much love I had for Jack. I rose, startled and energized, like I could repaint the interior of the house, clean every window, or run miles. Still tearless. Eyeing the empty hospital bed across the room, delivered and assembled just three hours ago, too late, I pointed with venom.

"I want that out of here. Now."

Steve, grateful for a distraction, jumped on it immediately. He retrieved his father's tools from the garage, and soon the bed lay in pieces in the driveway, awaiting pickup.

As a teacher, I'd stood before new students each fall with a list of classroom rules. Students half-listened, bodies wanting more sleep, brains blank, no questions, while I explained grading, expectations, and discipline. Rules made my classes safe and fun. Creating and following rules was second nature to me.

In "The Afterwards," as I came to call the days following Jack's last breath, life felt lawless and chaotic. In those days I craved structure, but I lost the ability to organize and plan.

"What do I do next, Jack?" My voice ricocheted loudly in the empty house.

The sharp jabs of raw grief folded me to my knees. I spiraled into confusion when I opened envelopes or file folders, watched words swim and meld together on the page, and put the contents down for later. I needed to fax information, find titles and account numbers, and read condolence cards. Too much, too much. I wanted everything to make sense when nothing did.

"What are the rules?" I pleaded with a good friend. She was the only one among my friends who had lost a husband. "How did you handle the holidays? What did you do with his clothes?"

Widowed in her late twenties, she had remarried and would soon celebrate a thirtieth wedding anniversary. She told me she honestly couldn't remember how she managed back then.

"What are the rules?" I yelled in frenzy to another friend on the phone, who had recently buried her stepfather. There was no good answer to my question.

For all the obituaries I had read about students' grandparents and parents, I had never studied them as a piece of literature. How was I supposed to compose this? How soon must I write and submit the obituary? What's the format? Should I include a picture? What facts should I include? What is the cost, and which newspapers? Jack was well known in multiple communities, between his sports officiating and teaching, old friends and new. There were many awaiting my words.

What are the rules for a "Celebration of Life?" A celebration for a man who was bigger than life? How soon after the death should it be? Do people eat there? What was I supposed to feed them? Did I have to write thank-you notes to the card senders? Expectations felt impossible to meet during this time of horrendous loss. A friend gave me an example of her stepfather's celebration program. I needed to design a program. There were speakers and picture boards. I needed to find a hall, pay rental fees, and decorate.

I learned that financial planners, real estate agents, and bankers had a rule for the bereaved: no major decisions in the first two years after the death of a spouse. What was "major?" Every decision seemed major. In the mornings, facing my closet and drawers, I wished an ensemble would fall out onto the floor so I didn't have to choose. I didn't care if buttons were aligned or colors coordinated. I wore the same clothes for several days in a row. Finding the energy to focus, select options, and execute demanded internal resources that were dwindling toward exhaustion.

It was a good rule, though. Don't sell the house, buy a new car, or give all the money away. A widow in a support group called it "widowed brain," when the thinking and memory worked poorly, stuck, revving in first gear on life's freeway. I stopped reading books because I forgot plots and characters from one night to the next. Starting chapters over again and again, I felt like I was slipping into Alzheimer's. Instead, I sought short articles in newspapers, magazines, and newsletters. I belittled myself over failing to hit "Start" on the microwave and the washing machine. *Come on, brain. Work!* I was totally unfit to make a major decision, or even a small one.

In a support group for the widowed, I met a woman whose wisdom helped slice a narrow path through the jungle of "The Afterwards." I had become so indecisive, distracted, and numbed. The teacher in me still wanted classroom rules; I wanted to know exactly how to live on.

"There are two rules for dealing with death and grief," my new friend told me. "Rule number one: People who love you, people who you love, should not die. Rule number two: If they should die, there are no rules."

Those were the only good rules.

Chapter 4
Unspoken: Words Not Said to Each Other

"Jack and I had a long conversation before he died," Mark said. "We talked for about forty-five minutes." His tone was casual, as if he were discussing his local Sedona weather.

My eyes widened and my body stiffened. As if someone had wrapped their arms around my ribs and squeezed the air from my lungs, I wheezed, "When?"

Mark was silent. Perhaps he heard the discord in my voice.

"When?" I demanded.

My voice was hard, nothing like the way I typically spoke to my favorite brother. After the torments and resentments of childhood passed, we had become dear friends. Our conversations were usually light, full of laughter and affection. But on this day the kitchen darkened, and my voice thundered back at me as if I stood in a tunnel.

"When?" One hand clenched the receiver hard while the other grasped the dark green countertop, steadying me. My feet lost the feel of the oak hardwood floor beneath me. I was sinking, standing on wet sand in a receding tide.

"A couple of days before he died," Mark said. "I think you were out walking the dog."

"What did you guys talk about?" My voice quavered. What did Jack say?

Mark paused. "At first, it was typical guy bullshit. Then I pressed him. 'I'm not going to ask how you are. That's sort of obvious. So tell me what it's like to be dying.' He cried, and I cried. He told me words that I will carry with me for the rest of my life. It totally changed me."

"What did he say?" I needed Jack's words to fill in the hole in my heart, the gap between us.

Mark was busy at work and needed time to recall the details. He said he would write it down in an email later. He ended the call, muttering an apology.

I hung up and pondered why Jack talked to Mark about death but not to me. Maybe I didn't ask the right questions. Maybe if I had asked something beyond, "Need a pill?" "How about some Jell-O?" "Gotta go to the bathroom?" "Got some emails? Want to hear 'em?" Maybe I would have had that forty-five-minute, life-changing conversation.

Weeks after Mark's revelation, other family members relayed their private conversations. Jack called his father three days before his death, and his son the night before. Hearing about each profound interaction, I replied in a neutral voice to protect my family from my outrage.

"How nice."

My glare burned into the walls, and my limbs rattled with rage. Damn you, Jack! What about my farewell chat? I was right here! What about me?

"I got nothing," I yelled to my therapist in my weekly session. "Not one single word."

"It was unfair. Time for some anger work," Kate said.

Down in our basement, two floors below our bedroom, I followed Kate's instructions. My anger slammed into a pillow on the guest room bed.

Damn you, damn them.

I thrashed the pillow for those who visited, for his three phone calls to family.

Enough strength, enough voice for your father, Steve, and Mark, but not for me? I struck the pillow. What do I have as our last conversation, Jack? Fuckin' zero!

Pound the pillow, pound the pillow.

Our bedroom, bathroom, and my adjacent study were on the lofted second floor above the open living room. The warm summer days sent the heat upstairs, and both rooms had small fans running, filling the rooms with a hum. When I stood at my desk, I had an easy view of Jack and could hear every moan and rustling of sheets. I downloaded and printed daily emails to be read aloud and made a list of friends who requested visits. On Jack's nightstand was a landline phone, its ringer turned off. The red message light occasionally flashed. Down fourteen tan-carpeted steps to the kitchen phone, I listened to phone messages, called back if necessary, checked the calendar on the wall, and used his red pen to write the visitor's name and time before heading back up the stairs.

On a medium-sized dry-erase board by the bed, a board I once used in my school office, I noted the visitors and arrival times in a fat purple pen, written large enough so Jack could read it from the bed without his glasses. When visitors arrived, I would stir him from sleep. I limited the daily number of visits and monitored their lengths, becoming not only a caregiver but also, begrudgingly, an administrative assistant and gatekeeper.

Disoriented from longer naps and stronger pain meds, eventually morphine, Jack often woke with a start; his eyes popped open. With his head on the pillow he asked the same questions: "What day is it?" "What's the time?" With the passing days, the eyes and voice became smaller. I checked the backlit clock, borrowed from a friend whose mother had Alzheimer's. The clock kept track of the passing time: the seconds I desperately wanted to slow down so I could have him with me longer, and the seconds I desperately wanted to run faster so his painful battle would be over.

"Oh, Jackson, you only slept two hours. It's a little after ten o'clock in the morning and still Tuesday," I answered in a soothing voice, putting down my book. I wasn't really reading a book, more like one page over and over.

"Do you need any water? Jell-O? Gotta go pee?" I rose from my chair, placed my hand on his bony shoulder, *Where did all your muscles go?* and kissed his smooth, warm head. I miss kissing lips. After final radiation for the brain tumors, completed six weeks ago, his entire head was hairless. I miss your silver hair, Bubba. I saw the blue, worm-like paths of veins on his skull, and my gut turned. This wasn't really him anymore. I turned away from him.

"It's okay, go back to sleep, Bubba," I whispered to an already sleeping man.

The midafternoon visitors came and knocked softly.

"Welcome, boys," I greeted them at the front door. Annie B gave a small bark at the strangers in her house, and I shushed her. Turning back to Malcolm and Bill, I said, "Ten minutes and he'll be tired. You'll see it."

Malcolm and Bill were softball officials who guided both our careers as umpires. Malcolm was a tall, slender man with a full head of silver hair who worked Division I college softball. Nothing ruffled his feathers on the field or off. Shorter and stockier than Malcolm, Bill was somewhere between a white-collar manager and a cowhand, a down-to-earth people handler. He smoothed the tough and argumentative Division I college coaches with his quick wit. He had the voice of a smoker, and at any moment, I expected to see chewing tobacco spit fly from his mouth. But he didn't smoke or chew. Everyone in the softball community loved and respected both men.

"How are you doing?" Malcolm slid his arm around my shoulder and pulled me into his side.

I let my shoulder lean into his chest and put an arm around his waist. When was my last hug from Jack? Weeks? Months? My chest stirred, feeling Malcolm's warmth, when I wanted Jack's.

"I'm okay." I pulled away and briefed our friends on what they were about to see: Jack hairless, skin hanging loosely on his once-muscular frame, his spark and laughter gone. They would have to look hard to see the Jack Reynolds they knew.

At the top of the stairs, both men stopped. The door was closed. Annie B had ascended the stairs ahead of us and sat at the bedroom door. About a week ago, Jack had requested that Annie B and I sleep elsewhere; we restricted his movement as he struggled to find comfort, especially Annie B, who loved to snuggle into his legs. On the floor of my study was an unmade blow-up single mattress, and both men flashed a look at it, then at me, as they waited to enter the bedroom. My eyes said, *Yes, guys, that's where I sleep. Pitiful, huh?*

I opened the door, and Annie darted to the bed, nestling against her sleeping best friend. Her eyes sent a dark challenge my way, warning me not to drag her off again.

"Jack?" I touched his shoulder. "Malcolm and Bill are here."

Jack exhaled loudly and turned on his back, which pushed Annie B onto the vacant side of the bed. She gave a small growl and settled in. His eyes opened slowly, and he greeted the two men with a weak, "Hi."

I grabbed the water glass with the straw, cradled Jack's head in my hand, and, after his long draw of water, I pulled a second pillow out and propped up his head. Both men stood and stared down at Jack until Bill broke the silence with his usual exuberance.

"Hey, big fellow," he said, like greeting an old drinking buddy in the local tavern. He rolled right into familiar talk about tournaments, teams, and coaches.

He paused for Jack to peep out, "Yeah, I remember him... What a fun tourney."

Suddenly, in one swift move, Bill lowered himself onto the bed and pulled Jack up to a sitting position, flinging Jack's legs over the side of the bed. Bill began to massage Jack's shirtless shoulders and back, the heel of his hand pressed deeply into the loose skin, continuing to jabber about his house remodel. My eyes bugged wide. Jack, you didn't cry out sitting upright like when I pull you up. Does this hurt? Jack had never asked me for a massage, and I never offered. Should I have been giving him massages all this time? Would that have helped with the pain?

Jack shot me a look. It meant something, but I didn't know what. Was I supposed to stop Bill's attempt at helping?

Damn, tell me, Bubba, tell me what to do.

My eyes shifted from Bill and Jack on the bed to Malcolm, who stood facing the backs of the two men. Tears streamed down his reddened face, and his hand was over his mouth to muffle any sound. I swallowed hard and gazed into the other room. Malcolm understood this was his last visit with his friend.

Bill finally stopped. He placed Jack's head back on the pillow, rose from the bed, lifted Jack's legs, and slid them under the covers. Malcolm pulled a handkerchief from his pocket, dried his face, and came around toward Bill and me.

"Take care." Both men tapped Jack lightly on the back to say goodbye. They did not say, You'll beat this, or See you back on the ball field soon.

Jack mumbled, "Thanks, guys." He rolled onto his left side.

At the front door, both men hugged me.

"Take care, Tally."

My tears came as I walked back up the stairs to Jack. With a deep breath at the landing, I dried my eyes and walked the last seven steps to the bedroom. At his bedside, I touched Jack on his bare shoulder and said, "That was nice to see Malcolm and Bill, wasn't it?"

Jack murmured, with his eyes nearly shut, "Is that the last one?" Thick fatigue filled his voice. Visitors didn't know what it took for him to be with them.

"No more," I said. I, too, felt exhausted, the space between my ribs hollowed out.

"Good." Jack, thoroughly spent, grew silent and still. I leaned over, kissed his head, and said, "I will always love you." My pet phrase, taken from a Dolly Parton song. I'd said these words to him for so many years, with every kiss.

I miss the tickle of your moustache.

At the foot of the bed, I rolled my tense shoulders and wished I'd gotten the rubdown. I recalled seeing Malcolm's grief as it mixed with my own. I listened to Jack's breathing. He winced occasionally as he shifted to find a more comfortable position. I cried quietly. What about me, Jack? No words left for me?

The resentment gnawed: our visiting friends robbed me of his precious time and energy. Thieves.

I dragged a growling Annie B off the bed, and she nipped at my hand. She'd been nestled into Jack's legs. Once both of us were out of the room, I closed the door behind us. She whimpered at the door, so confused. "Sorry, Annie B," I said and patted her head to go downstairs, hoping she would head to her heated bed by the kitchen. Once she was asleep there, I would return to my chair.

People assumed that Jack and I, together all day and night in those last months, talked plenty, bantered back and forth, sat with memories, laughed, and cried about lost dreams. We did have words, but it wasn't what they thought. We never had the kind of heart-to-heart exchange that sums up a life or honors decades spent together. Not even, *Thank you for marrying me.* I would have carried words like these with me for the rest of my life. Mostly, toward the end, we shared silence.

The night before his death, our final conversation focused on what would be his last trip to the bathroom. Due to the tightness in Jack's "Buddha Belly," sitting upright and standing to get out of bed caused him to groan and shudder.

He needed my help to get to the bathroom, and I needed his cooperation for our routine. That night, he didn't want to wake up long enough to go.

"Five more minutes," he begged, and fell back asleep. When I returned, I heard, "Another five, please," and another, and another, and another, while my patience became thin. Instead of sharing profound words, on our last night together, I struggled to get my husband out of bed and into the bathroom.

With a stomp of my foot, I demanded, "Now. No, don't go back to sleep. Now. It's late, Jack. I'm tired, too. Now. Please. I know it hurts. It won't take but two minutes, and you'll be back in bed. Now."

Silence.

We were alike. I held unspoken words, too. I can pinpoint the moment when I stopped being open, started picking my words carefully, and began to hold back information. The free-flowing tap of our easy conversations narrowed, became less spontaneous, more calculated. Instead of his friend and confidante, I became a shield between the reality of Jack's cancer and the remote hope that medical science could save him. He heard what I told him and read what I gave him.

On that fateful Friday four years ago, when the biopsy report revealed melanoma, the doctor gave us a terse instruction before sending us home: "Do not do any internet searching over the weekend."

Under her white jacket, her shoulders slumped like ours did, as if the news burdened her, too. She had gray hair and deep lines around her mouth; I imagined that she delivered such news to many patients, watching their eyes become teary or glazed over in disbelief. The doctor's gray eyes were clear and pointed, moving back and forth between us and the notepad on her lap. I shot a look at Jack, who had found something on the floor to hold his gaze. Scream with me, Jackson. Say something. But he held it all in.

"Sit with the shock; let it settle in," the doctor advised.

I heard her voice as if she were standing down a long hall, not in this white-walled, sterile room, where the overhead fluorescents seemed to dim, oxygen leeched out through the walls, and the ceiling crept downward.

"The appointment with the surgeon is Monday morning," she continued.

I processed this slowly: she had already made the appointment for us. When does a general practice doctor make an appointment unless it is very urgent?

My ribs seemed to press inward, crowding out the air left in my lungs. I ached for an escape, imagined darting out of that room through the white metal door, down the hallway, past people flipping through worn magazines in a waiting area, and out the glass front entry to the outside, where I could draw breaths of fresh air like a marathoner at the finish line. Only I would keep running.

Jack and I had different means of letting the diagnosis "settle in" that evening. Coming home from the doctor, we both changed from our work clothes into sweats and soft shoes. I fed Annie B and took her for a quick walk, then joined Jack in the daylight basement. The winter sun had set, and the room was lit only by the glow of the television in the corner. I turned on the light by the treadmill. Jack and his shock had settled in on the Lazy-Boy loveseat with the yellow and maroon pattern, which we'd chosen only for its sale price, not for its beauty. He was already lost in some CSI-lawyer series. I sat down next to Jack and held his hand, which was noticeably stiff with fear. After a few minutes, I found the sound of the television too loud, the scripted conversations too fake. I couldn't pretend to enjoy this façade of people having a normal day without cancer.

I went upstairs to the office and turned on the computer. My future, which had felt unencumbered a mere four hours earlier, lay crumbled on the floor of that doctor's office. I didn't know how shattered our lives were, or if they were repairable, but I needed to understand this sudden intruder, this cancerous third person in our marriage. The computer sounded its familiar start-up chord, and I jumped in surprise. I sat down with a prayer.

Oh God, I want this to go away. Stop it, please.

I Googled the medical term for skin cancer. I had forgotten the term the doctor used, but it popped up immediately. Where to begin when there were over twelve million hits for "melanoma?" Open, look, skip. Open, read, and write down words and phrases:

Oncology
Interferon
Stem-cell treatment
Immunology

Open, read, and cry. Of those twelve million hits, I read general information sites, searched for possible treatments using language I did not understand, and visited melanoma chat rooms. Once I'd scrawled out four pages of notes and questions, I caught my breath and dried my eyes. I closed my research and went downstairs to be with Jack.

"What were you doing?" he asked when I plopped back down beside him on the couch. Our eyes locked for a moment before he returned to his TV show.

After twenty-two years of marriage, he knew exactly what I was doing.

"Just reading," I said. I took his hand and pretended to watch TV. I never told him what I learned that night. That's when my silence began.

By Monday morning, I had read well over fifty articles. I knew the survival statistics for each of the stages, not yet knowing which stage described Jack. I'd given myself a preview of the forthcoming hell.

During the years ahead, in various phases of remission and relapse, I tried to get Jack to talk about life and death with me. I wanted to share an existential, philosophical discussion. After a positive report, tumors not growing but shrinking, I thought Jack might be receptive.

What do you believe happens to your spirit when your body dies? Is there a God? What was your purpose on this earth? How do you want to be buried and celebrated at the end?

Dissatisfied with his shrugged shoulders and nonchalant responses, I pushed a little harder, incredulous that my partner had never pondered the end of his life.

"Surely you've thought about death. I have."

No response.

"You know, just because you had this scare doesn't mean you will die first."

End of conversation.

I tried again. "I drive a longer distance than you for work, which means a greater chance of a fatal crash. In a way, you're lucky. You know the cause of your death. No surprises. Time to plan and think about it, Jack. Time to put your life in order. Some people don't get that."

At this, his eyes darkened, red racing from his neck up to his ears. His lips pushed into a thin line beneath his mustache. He stormed from the room, and I stood in the silence.

I tried humor, calling after him.

"There's always the proverbial piano falling out of the window and getting me first!"

At that, Jack grunted a chuckle but said nothing.

I stopped asking. Did I want to waste time, whatever was left, with anger, silence, separation, and resentment? What was most important was staying peaceful and connected. The falling piano became a joke between us, a cause of death we preferred to cancer.

I did not get the dialogue I craved. Jack's feelings stayed locked within him. I must live with never expressing mine.

As promised, Mark emailed me with Jack's final words to him. I recall printing the email, reading, and rereading it. But in those first years after Jack's passing, my sorrow jumbled details, erased entire weeks, and crumbled memories into dust. After that cherished page was lost in a move, I dug through boxes and rifled through files. I desperately called my brother, but by then he had only a murky sense of his conversation with Jack. Perhaps these were not my words to keep.

After twenty-six years of partnership with Jack, and several widowed years alone to reflect, my sense of his silence has evolved. Jack never talked to me about dying and death because he was afraid of facing failure. He was ashamed that he did not beat cancer.

When I reconstruct our moments together in those last years, in doctors' offices, in car rides to and from treatment, over restaurant tables, and in our home, I look for Jack's eyes meeting mine. I rarely find them. Jack couldn't meet my gaze at the end, not for long, because he carried his sorrow behind those gray-blue eyes. More than anything else, he wanted to save me from witnessing his decline, which he could not control. As a good husband, he wanted to stay by his wife's side and protect her. To his last breath, he was trying to do just that.

I'm okay with how things ended, Jackson, now that I've had time to think. You simply did your best. I doubt I will do much better when it's my turn to leave this Earth.

Whatever is ahead for me, it had better not be that damn piano that takes me out.

Chapter 5
Erasing: The "Business of Death" Burdens

The empty closet hangers were wire skeletons amidst the still-hung dress shirts and suits. Jack's winter jackets left his closet first, a horrific task that fall after his death. I could not justify my attachment to them when people would be cold and needy that winter, and we both believed that our blessings must be shared. Holding each tightly to my chest, I recalled dates, adventures, walks, and remodeling projects when I could see him wearing them. Some would be shipped far away, to his mother's Blackfoot reservation in Montana. Sweatpants, polo and T-shirts, socks, and underwear would go to a Seattle men's shelter. The dresser drawers we shared became half-vacant, too.

His dress clothes stayed with me, mementos to be swooped up when I needed him, crushed against my chest and face to inhale his scent. Eventually, I knew that his cologne would fade from the cloth, and I'd go straight to the bottle to retrieve the familiar lime smell, double-checking the cap weekly, terrified that the next time I sought this comfort, the contents would vaporize along with the memories. In a visual sweep of the house, there seemed to be less of him here. He stopped living with me.

I was unable to use any logic when I evaluated Jack's possessions. All of them became valuable. I kept a note with a useless phone number in his illegible handwriting, a "Life is Good" baseball hat with wiggly lines of his dried sweat on its brim, and a gnawed-on pencil. I snatched Jack's things from the hands of friends who tried to help me pack his possessions when they assessed something as Goodwill or trash-bound, with a disdainful look of *"You just don't get it."*

I picked something of his up, anything and everything, and held it like a fine champagne glass. I gingerly found a safe place to keep each treasure. Where to put his reading glasses? Should I leave the last books read on his bedside stand, or return them to the shelves in his study? Where is a safe place for his wallet? I put away some of his items. Into the dishwasher went the last bedside drinking glass he touched. Clothes that I washed before he died were finally folded and tucked into his dresser or into the piles to be given away. But the dirty clothes in the hamper remained untouched. They radiated the sweat of a man who once lived.

Throughout the house, something felt cockeyed, at times, downright eerie. Cool air tingled the fine hairs of my arms when I walked into the kitchen or stood by his study. I checked windows and doors, expecting one to be ajar. None were. The chill sank into my bones when I stood before the watercolor painting that we bought in Cannon Beach for our twenty-fifth wedding anniversary. Nothing had changed, but everything had changed.

My friends would think I was mad if I told them of his spectral visits, how his lime-scented aftershave floated into a room to let me know he was near. It was comforting that Jack was checking on me, "*I'm doing OK, Bubba,*" but unnerving that I could not put my face into his neck and inhale that smell off his body.

"What is going on?" I asked the walls.

Sounds became so loud after he died, as if rooms were emptied of furniture and carpet and walls were made of steel. The shuffled footsteps on the wood floor, the mishandling of forks, pens, and screwdrivers as they slipped from my hands and bounced a dissonant chord off the countertops or floors. Even the off-and-on light switches snapped louder.

I cocooned from outside intruders, neighbors, friends, and delivery personnel. I jumped as if struck from behind by the jolting assaults of the clang of doorbells, knocks, and phone calls. Often, I wanted to scream, "Go away! Go away!" to those who loved me.

Death turned up the volume.

In the dark, I heard footsteps on the carpeted stairs toward my bedroom. My heart and breath quickened. I pulled the blanket up, wanting to duck under, but I didn't. My eyes widened, anticipating a man's silhouette in the doorway. I waited and waited. Was this wishful thinking, or fear? I was tormented and wide awake, only to see nothing.

In the cool morning light, I woke on my side of the bed, the left side, and turned my head to see the flattened sheets on Jack's half. I ached for his warmth, to hear his snores and his grunt as he stirred under my touch. To hear, "Good morning, Talle."

But his body was taken by death months ago. The sounds of his existence were fading in my mind.

A few months before his death, I laid a tape recorder on my lap, tucked under the table, as we worked an easy Sudoku together. Jack never knew of the recording. I feared that he would think it was morbid or that I'd given up hope, but I was preparing for a day without him.

I never played the tape; I was scared of what I would hear, recalling our last game when Jack's eyes and voice were flat, shoulders drooped, as his cancer-ridden mind stumbled over an obvious answer. This was the man with his master's in education, who loved the History Channel, and who was unable to play a simple game. After he went to bed that night, I came back to the table and finished the game alone through tears and realized that I had lost my playmate.

I tried to record our last drive to the cabin. I hoped the recording would capture what we called "news broadcasting," when Jack and I would dance between topics while traveling, reporting, listening, settling into a comfortable silence, only to break it with another, "Oh! I didn't tell you about what happened on Thursday." The recording failed: the engine noise overwhelmed our voices.

I knew Jack's voice would be the first to leave: the brain cannot keep alive a sound that's not heard regularly. A widow told me she bought a new cell phone after her husband died because he left a message a day before his death, his last "I love you." I wish I weren't so compulsive, so tidy; I always erased his messages after listening. Now I couldn't change the outgoing message on the house answering machine because Jack's voice was on it. His voice implied, *There's a man in this house.* Not a woman alone, a woman afraid of the dark." When I wanted to be near Jack, I pressed that button to hear his voice in thirty-one words:

"You have reached the home of Tally, Jack, and Annie B. Reynolds. Please leave your name, phone number…"

The outside had become too loud and fast-moving. Trips to the store were short and completed with laser focus on a numbered list. There was no more meandering, lingering in the aisles to find new products, or stopping to see what fruits had come into season. I feared bumping into a neighbor, seeing the scrutiny in their eyes as they noticed I'd lost too much weight, as I fumbled for an answer to the question, *How are you doing?*

"The Business of Death" required that I tie up loose ends, but there was no pretty ribbon to tie around this process. I had new responsibilities as a widow, duties that called for standing in lines, facing strangers, and saying, "He has passed," again and again to people who could not know how much those words sting. After the burial, my attention was turned to matters involving lawyers, accountants, managers, government agencies, and front desk personnel. Like a fast-growing vine, the pile grew across the dining room table and cascaded onto the floor. Jack was still here, in name, on bills, bank statements, his will, and his death certificate. He was present in magazine subscriptions, professional newsletters, junk mail, and requests for charitable donations. I created a printed, signed response, "I need to inform you that Jack R. Reynolds died. Please delete his name from your records," and stamped return envelopes. A friend picked up his mail, needing notification. Bless her, one less task for me.

Vehicle registration was my first stop. I needed to become the sole owner of Jack's Ford truck, and the tabs were due. At the Department of Licensing, I pulled number "27" when "12" was up. Fifteen minutes later, I rose from the cracked vinyl seat and crossed the worn floor to the chest-high counter.

I'm sorry, Bubba, I gotta have my name on that title.

The harsh office lighting filtered through me into the hollowness within. I wanted to get this over as quickly as possible and then dash to the privacy of my car. I often cried while driving or in the shower, as if, oddly, being enclosed in glass was the safest way to be alone. Tears waited in the back of my eyes.

I shared a flash of eye contact with the middle-aged woman behind the counter, then diverted my eyes down. "I need to drop my husband's name from the title, add mine, and pay the tabs." I inched the title change form, our marriage license, and my legal name change documents across the counter. I garnered the strength to whisper, "He has passed."

Before his death, whenever we left the house, I carried Jack's DNR form (*Do Not Resuscitate*) in my purse. It was a God-awful chartreuse-colored document that beckoned his limited earthly time. A copy was stapled to the wall outside our home's front door in case I should ever call EMTs. If the DNR form marked the beginning of a detour in our lives, it was the death certificate that marked the fork in the road where Jack went one way and I another. I despised these two documents. They sent chills down my hands whenever I pulled them from the plastic folder I kept in the back seat of the car. Jack was gone, but these forms were still alive with purpose. Always with me.

The clerk's blue eyes softened as she peered over her gold-rimmed reading glasses to meet my gaze. With a sigh, she said, "Ms. Reynolds, I need a copy of the death certificate."

Trapped. I could not complete the business here without it. My insides felt like a street musician's six-instrument contraption with drums, harmonica, and bells, each with a different tune and beat, loud and jarring. The noise drowned out clear thinking. Unzipping the folder with shaky hands, I pulled out the certificate. Handing it over to her, I saw the blue, ornately edged stationery, knowing somewhere on it was his name, the date, and the cause of death. I diverted my vision to focus on a gray filing cabinet behind her, then a clock on the wall beyond. Anything but that death certificate. "Cause of Death" dissolved any illusion that he was just out somewhere and would be home soon. He was dead. There was the proof.

The woman left her chair to make a copy of the certificate. I stood with the hum of lights overhead, feeling the room shrink around me. Returning, she inked a rubber stamp, pressed it to the photocopied certificate and form, and stapled them together.

She pushed the originals back to me and asked, "Did Jack have a community property agreement? I need that, too."

I heard the past tense, *did*. The word rang in my mind: *did... did... did.* Past tense meant he was truly gone.

Nooooo, you're wrong!

I took a breath to settle back into the job at hand.

Focus.

"It's a community property state," I argued, knowing that the document she wanted was in a file marked "Wills," sitting on the dining room table at home.

I wanted this task checked off my long list. I wanted to grieve another loss, his barely readable yet so familiar signature on the title, which would disappear and be replaced by mine. One more erasure of proof that he existed with me.

Give me a frickin' break, I wanted to yell. I wanted to throw down the "widow card," get her to pity me enough to say, *I'll do it for you just this one time.* But I had so little energy and had spent too much on this errand already.

Damn you, Jack. Why wasn't my name on the title when you bought the truck?

I drove home, squeezing the steering wheel, and swore with each passing mile. I slammed the car door, grabbed the forms, and drove back. After a short wait, I stood before the same clerk and handed her the legal document.

"I'm so sorry for your loss," she said.

Not wanting to see the sincerity in her face, I diverted my eyes to the floor and whimpered, "Me, too."

She apologized for the hassle, and I thought, *It's not you. It was Jack's stupidity in the first place.*

With the new title ordered and tabs paid, I added the community property agreements to the document folder in the car. I put my sunglasses back on to shield my eyes from those caring souls who might stop me in the parking lot and ask, *Are you alright, dearie?*

I waited until I could clearly see the lines of the parking lot again, then started the car.

Please, JR, no more surprises. I can't take much more. I'm cracking.

At the bank, I needed to remove his name from the joint accounts and add a new beneficiary. A teller directed me away from the front counter to a waiting area. I sat in one of four black vinyl lobby chairs, watching others do their banking. A worker in paint-stained overalls cashed his weekly check; a mother with a child on her arm fussed with deposit slips. People glanced at me, then away, as if I didn't belong here. I felt like a misbehaving student, waiting for the principal to return to administer my discipline. I could hear my heart beating in my ears. I prayed for a speedy transaction. I prayed that I would not have to say anything twice or louder. One time was enough. Finally, summoned to a desk, sitting before a young assistant manager, the forms began their slide across the desk. I signed, he signed, boxes were checked, and copies were made. It was done so quickly, I was stunned: Jack was no longer a customer of this bank.

The credit card company was a different story. I added Jack onto my credit card after we got married, a man who lacked a sufficient credit score after he divorced his first wife. Over the years of bank acquisitions, someone had erroneously shifted my status from "applicant" to "co-signer," which meant the card was his. I discovered this when I called to drop Jack's name from the account. The company required me to close the account and reapply for a new card in my name. I lost my credit history and, the final sting, the credit limit was lowered by five thousand dollars. It was my card! I needed to pick a fight.

"Are you saying that after thirty years of paying on time on this account, I will have a lower credit limit?" I asked. "This doesn't have anything to do with me being a..." I stumbled over my words, mid-argument, "a single woman now, does it?"

Single woman tasted bitter in my mouth. It was so foreign to describe myself that way. There was silence on the other end of the line.

"Well, does it? Do you think that I will whip out that Visa card and spend money recklessly because I am widowed?"

Gripping the phone tighter, I had one more arrow to shoot. "Am I less financially responsible because there is only one name, and not a man's name, on the account?"

Silence.

The woman finally said, "Would you like to speak to a supervisor in the customer service department?" The offer meant I'd be placed on hold and listen to some gawd-awful music, tell the whole story again, and do what felt like begging for what was rightfully mine.

"No." I felt the fight drain out of me. "I'll call another day."

Hanging up, I scoffed to the heavens, *Damn you, Jack. Damn it all.*

I now understand why the living dedicate park benches and etched walkway bricks, establish memorial scholarships, and purchase gravestones. Something must remain. Something that cannot be obliterated with a simple phrase: *He has passed.* With a swipe of a hand, like wiping down the chalkboards of my youth, I had cleaned a man's earthly slate. There was dust on my hands, proof of his life and my hand in his erasure. Some worldly possessions were passed on to me.

But there were treasures that couldn't become mine simply by signing a piece of paper. Jack had a superior recall of events. He could pull up names, dates, and specifics from thirty years back.

"Where did we have that amazing seafood dish in a bucket?" "Remember when we rescued that skier after seeing her butt sticking out of the snowbank? When was that?"

I relied on him to fill in the blanks of my poor recall. I lost rich stories, details of our years together. He took those with him.

When asked for marital status from here on, I will check "Single" or "Widowed" instead of "Married." When introduced at a party, "This was Jack's wife," I will inevitably think, "*No, I am his wife*". But I was not defined by that role anymore. I was no longer Jack's caregiver. With the passing of Jack's father, I was no longer a "daughter-in-love," his pet name for me.

I lost the marital vocabulary, once so fluid, the pronouns of "ours" and "we." From henceforth, it was "mine," "my," and "me."

Chapter 6
Envy: Seeing Other Couples

I hid in a place without phones, doorbells, or the *how are you doing?* Away from those who offered help or shared their tears with me. Away from my questions. I needed a place to walk where no one knew the whys of the reddened eyes behind my sunglasses. One month after Jack's death, and one week before his Celebration of Life, I returned to the Oregon Coast, our vacation spot for over twenty years. I'd paid the deposit eight months ago, when the cancer had not yet reached his brain, assuming his luggage would be in the car with mine.

I stayed in our motel, in the same room with its ocean view and a small kitchen. "I need only one key," I said to the kind woman at the front desk. My dog, Annie B, sat obediently by my side. The woman was older than me by a good fifteen years and stood taller, too. She knew Jack: he was usually the one who paid the balance, made a reservation for next year before we left, and chatted with her husband. Patting my hand that rested on the counter, she began to cry as I told the story of his passing. My tears edged my eyelids, and I could feel my knees beginning to wobble. *There is no place to hide.* Her warm hand rested on top of mine. *He touched so many who must touch me.* I slid my hand out from hers with a stale, "Thank you." As I turned to leave the office with my key and the dog, I paused to put my sunglasses back on.

My stay was Sunday to Wednesday, not the usual full week. Jack's Celebration of Life would be Saturday. I wanted to miss that, let them celebrate, eat the cake, talk about him, talk about us without me, watch the PowerPoint show I assembled of his life. But I would play the widow, sit in the front row aisle with Mark by my side, and feel eyes on the back of my head.

This was the first step, this coastal retreat, of thousands I would walk on a widow's path. I tried my best to relive our past vacations. In the summer sun, in shorts and a T-shirt, I walked the town but felt more repelled than invited into the familiar shops, art galleries, and restaurants. Those commercial doors seemed too heavy, stubborn as a "Pull" when it's a "Push."

An order of clam chowder at Bill's Tavern tasted like skim milk. A fantastic watercolor was washed with the grays of my mood. The rhythmic hum of the waves, the sweet, cool sea air that smelled of salted caramels, calls of the gulls floating up from the beach to the crowded sidewalks, nothing soothed. The sand filtered into my shoes, into my socks, gritty between my toes. I stopped often to shake out socks and shoes. Shake out the discomfort.

The noise of the town screeched in my ears like train brakes: babies flailing in parents' arms, whining children being tugged away from the doors of the candy shops, revving motorcycles carrying couples garbed in black leather. Even laughter irritated.

My favorite jog was along the water at low tide, which offered a wide margin of wet, firm sand. I wanted an easy, straight path. I wanted to run out my grief. Or was it "outrun?"

Instead, I was annoyed, sidestepping marooned jellyfish, broken sand dollars, strands of seaweed with sand fleas, and people with dogs. I wanted the shadow of Jack on the sand next to mine. With the sunlight still glimmering above the horizon and its band of fluorescent light on the sea, I sought the quiet of the room.

Drawn by the setting sun, tourists trekked down the sandy path adjacent to the motel to the ocean's edge. Pulled from the beachfront rentals and shops, with children and dogs in tow, arms of firewood, fancy cameras dangling from lanyards, they came to witness a day's end.

Jack and I were once among those beachside masses, beach chairs in hand, picking a spot to view the intense colors of the sunset. "Nothing tonight," we would sigh with disappointment when late afternoon clouds rolled in and blocked the display. We would return to the room and settle in with our newly purchased beach reads, watch an old movie, or catch a baseball game, nestled together on one of the queen beds.

Cancer treatment played havoc with Jack's internal thermostat. He chilled easily, and we relocated our sunset viewings to the indoor chairs. Without him now, I turned my swivel chair toward the west, anticipating that glorious sunset. My gaze fell upon an older couple straggling behind the crowd. They strolled with a slow gait, elbows interlocked for closeness, for mutual balance. Their stooped shoulders were wrapped in matching coats for the forthcoming evening's cool. Silvery white hair slipped out from the edges of his ball cap and around her knitted beret. Their heads tilted toward each other, much like two magnets ready to snap together as they walked on. Her free arm waved to emphasize some point in a conversation. With his head thrown back, he roared his amusement, loud enough for others nearby to turn back and look at him, smiling too. It's a private joke, I imagined, one to be told many times.

Tears dammed at the edges of my closed eyes, and my body collapsed deeper into my chair. The first reel of my mental movie of our senior years began to roll.

Jack has gone bald like his father, not from the chemo but from age. I stopped having my hair colored, let the salt and pepper take over. Our conversations are centered on comparing our aches, ailments, and new medicines. Jack's hearing loss has dictated my positioning; I stay on his left side. I foresee, after our joints demand a reprieve from heavy lifting and stairs, our move to a rambler-style home. Then, senior housing. To stay active, we pull the golf clubs out from storage.

Reel two is on the uptake:

Without him, I am alone. There is no one to accompany me to medical appointments, hear the results of tests, or provide reminders to take medications. I am alone when I awake from surgery. I am alone when I receive the bad news.

The movie abruptly ended, and, out there, I saw them still walking arm in arm. Within my gut, envy steeped like tea, darkening, then cooling, like the bite of a winter wind. Like a madwoman, I wanted to bolt out of my room, screech into their faces, *Why do you get more years than us? Why? What makes you two so special?*

My body ached for some wild movement to untie the snarl I was in. If I were a dancer, I might have known the right leaps, twists, and stomps to unknot myself. If I didn't respect the motel's owners, I would have thrown the glassware against the wall, shredded the towels, and blankets. Instead, grabbing the dog leash, I set out for a walk.

Couples were, are, everywhere. I hadn't noticed them when I was part of their clan, but after Jack's death, I became an outsider. My trip to the coast was the first of many such encounters. In grocery stores, my stares would pierce through older couples picking out tomatoes, pasta, and canned tuna for a meal. I would come to detest the duos holding paint color samples at home improvement stores, gut-punched when I heard, "What do you think of this blue color for the bathroom?"

I learned to avoid watching couples in restaurants, nibbling from each other's plates and saying, "Oh, you must taste this salmon!" The clinking of glassware as they toasted each other brought bile to my mouth. When they walked down sidewalks hand-in-hand, I endeavored to look away quickly. Their easy conversations. Their comfortable silences.

When friends announced wedding anniversaries and special milestones, I dragged out "Congratulations" with a plastic smile. But they heard no exclamation point in my voice. Envy drowned sincerity. They were good people, good couples, and I honored what it took to remain committed and loving to each other. But I was not wholly happy for them. I could not separate my widowhood from their marriages.

Someone had to be first among my crowd to lose their partner. My friends couldn't help that it was me. But in a dark corner of my soul, in a fleeting moment, I wished the hell of widowhood upon them. Let one of them sleep alone in a queen bed. Not me.

From here on out, it hit me differently when friends complained to me about their husbands, "He doesn't like to talk in the car, so I bring along knitting." Jack and I loved to drive together, babbling random thoughts, planning a remodel, exchanging trivial moments of our workdays. We called it "news broadcasting." Topics changed quickly, and neither of us had to comment on what the other said. Hearing my friend, I would imagine punching her husband hard in his gut.

The unspoken words would haunt you.

"I know he loves me, but his family never says it, so he never does," another friend told me at a café one day, where I sat frozen in my chair. Jack would say, "I don't love you. I adore you." Even when we had our angry words, stomping around the house, remaining on separate floors, and, if we passed in the hallway, trying not to let even our breaths touch, we called a truce with "I still love you."

"It's a marriage of convenience. I cannot live without his financial support," still another friend told me, describing her husband's affairs and how she remained loyal to the marriage. And yet, they were still coupled. And alive. My husband, with his own set of faults, was gone. A marriage of passion, companionship, and respect was over. It wasn't fair.

I carried on these imaginary conversations while walking the coastline. *If you don't treasure each day with each other*, I thought with venom, "*Trade places with us. You don't deserve more time.*"

The sky was turning into its evening colors: the once-bright blue overhead was brushed navy, and above the motel roof, I saw shades of pink and yellow on swirls of cotton-candy clouds. The cooling air teased the hair on my arms and legs.

I stopped in the middle of the sidewalk under a tall cedar tree and turned back to my trailing dog. Annie B was fifteen years old. Her strides were stiff and slow, and her nails occasionally scraped against the pavement, making a rasping sound. She once ran this beach for hours, chasing tennis balls thrown by Jack, catching some mid-stride and others out of the air. From a distance, she looked like an ebony hyphen dashing along the ocean's edge.

I felt another tug on the leash, signaling Annie B's resistance to the walk. With her sad eyes and slow tail wag, she told me, *I'm doing the best I can.* I bent down and kissed the top of her head.

"Me too, Ms. B. The best I can." We turned back toward our room and the sea.

Chapter 7
Forgotten: Forgetting A Sacred Date

The 28th crept in slowly, rippling chills over my skin even under a warm quilt. The date took up room in my thoughts, pushing out needed grocery items, names of neighbors' children, and the location of my keys and glasses.

"*Look at me*." The voice came from the kitchen, whisper-like. I stopped walking and turned. No one was there, of course, but my eyes were drawn to the wall above the phone cabinet, to the dry-erase calendar the size of a shoebox lid. I moved to stand in front of it and focused on a two-inch square in the last row of calendar days. I picked up a purple dry-erase pen and wrote "Jack's Day" within the square's thin black lines.

I held Jack's final day like a photo-album page, archived and studied. Jack's last words, the feeling of lying beside his chilling body. After his last breath and the arrival of the mortuary attendants, I could not watch his body wrapped in the teal sheets of our bed and carried from our bedroom; I escaped to sit on a basement stair two floors below. A friend who was with me yelled that the car was about to leave. I came upstairs to the front door and waved goodbye to the mortuary's SUV as it drove away.

On the 28th of each month, my eyes clouded over. I missed him with a passion that threw me toward the edge of insanity. Angst churned in my gut, an acid that burned. Sadness stiffened in my shoulders and neck. When the sadness reached my legs, tension left in a rush, and my muscles went slack until I was no longer able to stand

and slumped onto the floor. Again and again. Every month. Embedded in that day were the memories of the 28th of June when Jack died.

The day was a milepost marker between his death and the afterward of my life. What had I done from sunrise to sunset? Often, I couldn't remember, although the dirty clothes in the laundry bin, the newspapers in the recycle bin, the dog's full water bowl, and living plants inside and out were proof that I was here. Time simply moved on.

The 28th bit harder over time and clawed fiercely at skin that had thinned and scarred in the new solitude. Manic cleaning distracted me from reliving the anniversary: a shower door, the top of the refrigerator, or a bathroom drawer. Or I sank into the mattress, limbs weighted down by recollections, unable to stir up any hope in my dark hole. I never knew which extreme would overcome me. Deep sobs accompanied both and were always unexpected. Sometimes insignificant items triggered bouts: his unused toothbrush on the bathroom counter, a stray dirty sock in the laundry, or a telemarketer asking for "Mr. Jack Reynolds."

When the 28th arrived, emotions were dry and brittle like autumn leaves. Breath shallow. Foods in the pantry tasted unseasoned or stale. I forced something down only because I feared getting sick; the vision of being ill in bed, without anyone to bring me hot broth or lightly buttered toast, helped get something down my throat.

Of course, there was no need to mark "Jack's Day" on the calendar: living alone provided ample reminders of his passing. There were bills addressed to my name only and mail addressed to Jack that I had to open. Grocery lists lacked his beer, tortillas, and coffee. I could mix the newly purchased black bras and underwear, after tossing out the white ones, with my jeans, shorts, and T-shirts for a smaller weekly laundry load. His half of the bed, with its sheets still tucked in and pillow undented, told me I slept alone.

But I did mark that day. I needed him on the calendar, like an observer in absentia of what I am doing with my life. I wanted him here. The 28th was more important than anything else on that calendar: a soccer game, morning coffee with friends, or the aging dog's vet appointment.

Marking the monthly calendar was a time to hold a conversation with him. I would whisper to the wall, "I made it another month, Jackson. Alone. Who would guess?"

I did my chores and all of his, cleaning the toilets, vacuuming, and sweeping off the porch and deck. I was enduring far better than I imagined. I heard him say, "I never doubted that you could."

Eyeing a forthcoming theatre performance, our "date night" six times a year for more than twenty years, I whispered, "I will miss you in the chair next to me."

I promised my therapist that I'd make five phone calls before giving the tickets away. I detested my new "single" status, so I endured these calls to friends every two months or so to find someone to sit next to me.

Standing in the kitchen, I made my first call. "Hey, Katy, can you go with me to the theatre on Sunday, a 1:30 show?" No, she was busy with her sisters that day. "Next time," she told me. The phone got heavier. Sand was filling my brain. Before I made the next call, I wrote down a script with the day, time, and name of the show to avoid stuttering. I had four more calls to make.

"Denise, are you doing anything on Sunday afternoon? Got theatre tickets for Sunday's matinee, 1:30."

"Sorry," she said. She and her husband were heading to Canada to see some friends. "Call again," she said. Tears gathered. I wanted to throw the phone in a rage.

Damn you, Jack.

As I dialed the third friend, fatigue sneaked into my muscles until I had to focus to keep the phone in my hand. I wanted to place my head on the floor and rest. I waited while her phone rang. *Please don't answer; go to voicemail. I need a nap.*

Years before retirement from our jobs in education, Jack and I would start each month staring at the dry-erase board in our morning slippers and sweats. I'd have my activities in my PDA device and work calendar, while Jack's dates were scrawled in his left-handed scribble on an envelope of unopened mail.

"Let's start with this week. Any wrestling board meetings?"

"Oh, yeah. Got a letter last week," and he left for his study to retrieve it.

Drumming fingers on the countertop, I'd hear the envelope being ripped open and then a pause, as he would read it on his way back to the kitchen.

"Tomorrow night, 5:30. Dinner meeting. I'll go directly from school." This meant rearranging my afternoon to get home early for the dog's feeding and walk. I'd close my eyes and take a deep breath to melt the ice forming in my words.

"Anything else? Wrestling?"

"Yeah. Got a couple of high school matches this week and a tournament this Saturday." These were not in his envelope. He returned to his study for a printout of his officiating schedule. The sound of his printer starting up came down the hall into the kitchen.

I would wait, shaking my head in disgust at the wall, muttering, "You jerk, this doesn't have to be so hard or so slow." When he returned, I handed over the pen and left the kitchen on the pretense that I had a chore elsewhere in the house.

I was convinced we would avoid arguments if he only did it *my way*, writing it all on our calendar at the start of the month and updating regularly. Each month, the board became coated with "Where were you?" and "I'm sorry, I forgot to tell you," as tensions melded onto the white background of the calendar. Maybe if I'd just let Jack come and go, like a single man, without adhering to my need to know everything, maybe then I could stop watching the clock, go to bed, and sleep. But that wasn't me. When he didn't come home on time, I imagined scenarios: a car accident, a state patrol cop at the front door, and a frantic rush to a hospital ER. I wrapped myself in fear, and it escalated with passing hours. When he was home, I treasured his presence, even if he was downstairs watching TV and I was upstairs doing schoolwork. I wanted to be able to find him at any moment for a hug and kiss.

My calendar commitments were in my favorite color, blue, which left Jack the choice of red, green, orange, or purple in the five-pen pack. He chose red. Annie B got the orange, and our "date night" got green. The calendar was busy with rainbow notations of our lives, and the little squares did not contain enough space for all we did. We lived big, filled our weeks, and thrived in our passions and interests. As his cancer progressed, Jack's medical appointments in red dominated the calendar, often overflowing into adjacent days. The green pen sat in the cup, used less and less.

Readying the calendar for July, the first month without him, the initial task wasn't picking up the pen. It wasn't checking my phone's calendar. It was erasing June.

Erasing.

Erasing those red marks that recorded his final appointments, final visits from friends, final tasks that were once his but became mine. Once the board was wiped clean, I would never see his handwriting on the wall again. June was a visual diary of his last twenty-eight days. Henceforth, all the appointments and events on the wall would be in blue or orange. Just my life and Annie B's and none of his. I was deleting his existence further from this earth. All blue or orange. No red or green. I tasted the bitterness of being the survivor.

Bracing one hand on the wall, steadying myself, I gripped the blue pen. "Goodbye, Jack," I mumbled, wiping my eyes for focus. I dragged the eraser end left and right for the first slow, choppy strokes. The first week of June went by. Then another Sunday through Saturday cleared. The rumble of pain stirred within. *Don't stop*, I yelled to my hand, feeling the drain of momentum. *Keep going*! Downward, as if dragged through sand, left, then right, the eraser arrived at the last row, pausing before the 28th. *Do it!* My head yelled, but my heart said, *Give me a moment here. Let me honor his battle before letting go.* With a final quick swipe, eyes closed, I choked, "Goodbye, Bubba."

And the board was blank. My pain was unleashed, and I collapsed to the floor. Kneeling, rocking from the waist, I wept into the oak floor. The calendar was cleared for July.

In some cultures, red is the color associated with life. At Jack's Celebration of Life, I wore a red blouse with this very intention: one life spent, another life lives on. Initially, I thought the red pen might be appropriate to mark "Jack's Day" each month. Standing in front of the calendar, I selected red from the cup: his color, his pen. I remembered it in his left hand, his illegible writing, how often I had to ask, "What's this word?" But the red pen felt heavy as it hovered over the 28th. Returning his pen to the cup, I chose purple, the color of healing, a color formed by the combination of red and blue.

Chapter 8
When: Disposing of His Lasts Meals

The quiet was brutal without Jack.

For the last thirty days, all the sounds inside the house were mine and the dog's. No rattling of hangers, no wooden drawers being knocked in their frames. No aroma of brewed coffee to denote that he'd started his day. Annie B slept most of the day on the heated bed that soothed her arthritic hips, nestled into the new stillness.

I buried the vocabulary of cancer care and its medicine with Jack's passing: oncology, chemotherapy, radiation, neuropathy, amiodarone, metoprolol, senna, prochlorperazine maleate, and sulindac. When I opened the front door and pushed out hospice and morphine, the new words of the survivor came in. Awful words. I stammered over "his remains" and "Jack's body" when I dealt with the funeral home. I leapt past "He's dead" or "He's died" when speaking to others; those seemed to rhyme with "He's never coming back." Instead, I learned to use the more spiritual "He's passed on." Not "I am widowed." Never "I am a widow." That acidic noun stomped on "spouse" and "lover." I still thought of myself as Jack's wife.

In the pre-dawn light, I woke after a fitful night of sleep, peeked at his side of the bed, and whispered to his undented pillow, "I miss you so much." I yearned for *Good morning, Talle*, or a healthy snore as he turned over in bed and left the morning to me. I even craved, selfishly, a grunt of cancerous pain from that side of the bed, signaling that I was not alone.

Throughout the day, I repeated those words, "I miss you so much," to the artwork we bought, his favorite spot on the couch, the walls we remodeled, and empty spaces. This widow's chant.

From the top of the dresser, I grabbed the same gray T-shirt and shorts I wore yesterday. I don't remember when things were last washed, time was either slippery or stagnant, and I didn't care. Only clean underwear was mandatory. My sneakers, muffled by the carpet upstairs, scraped like sandpaper on the wood floors of the main level on the way to the kitchen.

I peeked around corners with anticipation of seeing him in his sweats, coffee mug in hand, and, with a broad smile, greeting me: *Mornin', Talle. I'm home*. But each room was empty, and I backed into my denial.

Through the kitchen's open windows, cooler air mixed with the heat still trapped inside from yesterday's summer day. The refrigerator's low bass hum joined the songs of morning birds. I don't know which song belongs to which bird, never retrieved the bird book, nor a good pair of binoculars to track the sources of the greetings. I wanted to address them by name, to have a conversation. But I only listened.

Annie B's fur was black down her back, with tan and white swatches on her sides and belly, and white-socked paws. She watched me as I watched her. Another sadness filled me as I eyed her white muzzle: it was once all tan. I know what I must do someday, alone. "I love you, Miss B." I leaned over to kiss her head, and a tear fell on her. She doesn't like crying, she was one reason I cried into a pillow, in the shower, or in the car, and she turned her head up and licked my face.

"Thanks, B. You're a good dog." Massaging her head, I wiped my face dry with the sleeve of my shirt.

Out the front door and down the patio stairs, I grabbed the poop-scoop shovel that leaned against the garage wall, an old round point with a fractured wooden handle held together with duct tape, and headed toward the cul-de-sac for her "morning duties." This was Jack's job. I remember watching them from the kitchen, the man and his first puppy, on this walk across the driveway to the street, with the shovel in his hand. Once back inside the house, he'd feed her, start his morning java, and our day would begin.

I miss you so much, I said to the heavens as Annie B and I took our first steps across the driveway in the morning air. *So much.*

Back inside, Annie B waited by her bowl under the big window. I let the kibble cascade slowly into her bowl, so as not to startle her or rattle myself.

I stood before the stainless-steel refrigerator, a concession to Jack's preferences during the remodel, with its metallic sheen like a shield, armor-like to protect something good to eat, something that would bring a tang to my taste buds, a comfort to my gut.

I lost my appetite, but I knew my body needed something. I ran out of milk a week ago for my routine breakfast of cereal and switched to toast and jam. The bread bag was in the recycle bin. Several days ago, the orange juice pitcher was washed and placed back in the cabinet. No fresh produce in the clear refrigerator bins or in the fruit basket on the counter. The shelves were barren of casseroles left in the early days, gifts from neighbors honoring the social obligation to the bereaved. They moved on with their lives, as if grief had a shelf life and it passed an expiration date.

I pulled open the door and stared in. The light from that single appliance bulb cast my thinning shadow into the room. I had already lost a pant size, inching down to another one. Worried friends asked, "What are you eating?" and shook their heads when I said, "Mostly popcorn."

The escaping refrigerated air pricked at my exposed skin as it escaped, taking some of my sleepiness with it. I could easily close the door and step back into the warmth of the kitchen, but I remained. The shelves and drawers, empty of anything for breakfast, stymied my thoughts. Sometimes it was too hard to decide to do anything other than remain upright and still.

I noticed the remaining condiments on the door racks, and my teary vision became a kaleidoscope. The yellows of mustards, reds of ketchup and salsas, greens of pickle relish and verde sauce twirled with each blink. My ketchup, his salsas. My relish, his mayo. So many meals together. Smells of quesadillas, marinara sauce, and hamburgers held inside each jar. The past spun in my mind until I felt dizzy. I could not slow the carousel of chaos. A blur.

I resisted leaving the house to shop for food. I didn't want to leave Annie B behind, and I didn't want to enter a grocery store to purchase single-serving items and microwave-quick meals. I didn't want the kindness of neighbors who would wave me down to ask, "How are you doing?" and "Can we help with anything?"

"OK," I'd tell them. "Thank you." "Nothing now." Five words, all truthful. I wanted to give them more, the caregiver in me wanted to soften their concerns, but since Jack's passing, I was overwhelmed. Five words were all I had.

I did not want the cashier to ask, "Did you find everything you needed?" and "How are you today?" Because the words "I lost my husband" always at the tip of my tongue, could tumble out to a stranger. Those four words chipped at my denial. If I said them enough times, it would make Jack's passing real. *He's really, really dead.* I struggled to distinguish one-dollar bills from fives and tens to pay the bill. I held on until I got to the car, shut the door, and dissolved.

I dreaded the inquiries from those who saw us as a couple: the barista at the local espresso stand, the waiters at the breakfast café and our favorite pho restaurant, the clerk at the drugstore, and the owner of the Baskin-Robbins who asked, "And where's your husband today?"

At the grocery store, I forgot whatever I didn't write down, and even then, I often overlooked an item, like milk for the cereal. I did without until I was forced to go back into the world with a new list. Often, I misplaced the list entirely and found myself in the middle of an aisle, stomping my foot and hissing, "So damn stupid," irate that I was unable to recall what I needed. I fumed around the store, hoping the sight of an item on a shelf would trigger my memory. Popcorn saved me on those days. I knew exactly where it was shelved.

On this warm summer morning, my right hand held the refrigerator handle, and the other hung weightless by my side. My feet glued to the light oak floor, and my eyes pulled to the back of the second shelf, where the gleam of plastic wrap flashed. Five glass bowls of Jell-O: three green, lime-flavored, and two red, cherry. Two of the bowls had bites missing, with spoons still in them. One sheet of Saran Wrap covered them all. These were the remains of Jack's last meals.

Closing my eyes, I saw it all again: asking him which flavors he wanted before heading to the store. Rushing through the grocery aisles and the express checkout. Speeding home, all the way with a plea,

"Please don't die before I get back." Heating the water, doing the quick preparation method with ice, watching him eat, only to placate the worry I wore. Hearing him say, "I'm done for now. I'll have more later," a refrain that came quicker with each meal.

Yesterday, I finished drinking the last opened bottle of mixed tea and lemonade. That quenched Jack's thirst until one day it didn't; only ice chips helped. Even after he stopped requesting the tea mix, I never sipped from it, thinking it could again become the drink of choice. I stocked it in the house, ready for him, everything always ready to give him comfort. Now the plastic bottle rested in the recycle bin. Another minuscule act of removing Jack from the house.

Two days ago, I felt the ire of seeing Jack's favorite carbonated drinks in the refrigerator: liters of Coke, ginger ale, and cherry-flavored soda water, alongside his lime-flavored Gatorade. Those useless drinks did nothing to extend his life. I didn't even flinch while I poured the liquids down the drain. I wanted to stuff the plastics into the disposal, pulverize them into little pieces, gather the remains, and burn them. Instead, with two hands and clenched teeth, I twisted the plastic bottles into skinny tubes before slamming them into the recycle bin.

But I will never eat the Jell-O. His last meals. I wish gelatin could evaporate, so that one day, opening the refrigerator, the glass dishes would be clear, spoons resting inside them. Vanished. How does one tell if the Jell-O is no longer edible? With a half-hearted chuckle, I created the criteria: when it molds. Maybe, with a white or blue crust, I will act.

The Jell-O became sacred, equal to many of Jack's possessions in the house: contents of his bathroom drawers, the books, cards, and glasses in his nightstand, clothes in the dressers and hung in the closet, in the dirty laundry, the tools, his truck, the chilled beer in the garage's little refrigerator.

I cannot move his things. I must keep everything in place exactly as it was on the day he died, in hope that he will return. What would he think to find the house half empty? What kind of wife was I to remove what was his before I am sure he was gone?

Chapter 9
Mirror: I Wish I Were a Better Caregiver

Several months after Jack's death, the silence pressed hard against me, and I wanted to push back, but it was like pressing into air. The quiet was here to stay. I leaned forward and rested my hands on the cool white tiles of the bathroom countertop, tiles chosen by me and placed by Jack. With a fingertip, I traced the grout line where it skewed.

I heard the tiles speak, "*Good enough.*"

Years ago, at the tile store, the tiles were laid out in the aisle: I would manipulate the pattern, step back, grab another contrast color, step back again, and evaluate. Repeat. Try again.

"Good enough," Jack said on the fourth variation, frustrated by my pursuit of perfection.

Only I knew that spot behind my faucet where he missed a small three-quarter-inch cut so that the grout line did not continue in a straight line but veered ninety degrees. Jack wanted to chisel out his error, but I was tired, and the tiles were firmly in place. We had started early in the morning, and a growl from my stomach demanded a late lunch.

"Good enough, Jack," I pleaded. "No one will know but us."

He conceded, although I saw a worry in his proud eyes that I might think less of his work, that I might think less of him.

In the bathroom, the dimmed bulbs in their cut-glass domes appeared like small tea candles on the wall. I observed myself in the mirror. The muted light left my brown eyes hidden, nearly black in their sockets; the dark circles underneath and the creases of stress in my forehead and around my mouth were softened. I pushed back my drooping shoulders, hearing my mother's harsh reprimand, *"You're slouching."* In my youth, her words would bolt me into a soldier-like stance.

"Good enough?" I asked the mirror. I turned and left before I could hear *"No."*

With its farewell, cancer presented a new mirror, and I peered into the glass. I saw images tucked into dank corners and behind drawn curtains, memories I preferred forgotten, not relived. That mirror stripped me of the illusion that I always did my best, that I was more than good enough, that I walked into widowhood as an innocent bystander and dedicated caregiver. In that glass reflection, I saw images of my regrets, my list of everything I "should-have-could-have-but-didn't," the moments when I had a choice to act with compassion, tenderness, and patience, but I ran or hid instead. Those memories crept out in the days that I was tired and had little resistance.

For some time, I avoided my reflection. I played a poor game of hide-and-seek, like the parent who tells the child, *"I'll be 'It.' You hide."* Once the child leaves the room, the parent quietly returns to a book. The child has no option but to remain still and hidden, to mark time. I sent my failures away to hide, promising to face them later. I was the seeker who did not seek. The passage of months seemed to make my demons bolder; over time, those horrid creatures peeked out frequently, even taunted, *"Here I am. You are stronger now. Come find me."*

And eventually it was true. I was strong enough, and the hideous feeling of guilt became too much. Maybe the glass would only reflect who I was: overstressed, overtired, and overworked. I was so frightened to witness life slipping out of Jack's body, one exhale at a time. His longer naps, lack of appetite, and fewer words showed he was separating from me, regardless of how close or how long I sat in the chair next to the bed. But Jack's "No! No!" crept out from deep within. I didn't want those demons hidden anymore. *"Come on out."*

The truth is, I was selfish. One of my greatest worries was imagining the day Jack was gone. Everything, house care and maintenance, finances, dog care, cabin would become all mine. I would be forced to live alone. Could I do it? That question, like a curious cat, slinked around my steps and through my thoughts during Jack's long periods of sleep. In the silence, I walked through rooms and hallways, stood before the watercolor art that we bought, the walls with new lights and color, and sat on one of the two breakfast stools in the refinished kitchen. Piece by piece, we had created this home, so full of his booming voice, our giggles, and our shared dreams. With his death, could I live in this stillness and vacancy and not go crazy?

The truth is, I was cowardly. I prayed for Jack's final gasp of air to be at 2 a.m., muffled, so as not to stir me from sleep. Was my rest more important than being awake at his side at the end? The day we learned that the cancer had reached his brain, with the possibility of a stroke, I begged my God to take all of Jack and protect him from a life with a partially functioning body and mind. I didn't want him to suffer, but I also didn't want to deal with all that is needed after a serious stroke: bathing, feeding, and, worse, cleaning him. Would God hear my petitions for Jack to slip away while I walked our dog, detained a few minutes in the cul-de-sac because a neighbor stopped for an update? Was it wrong to selfishly relish the attention when the neighbor focused on me for a few moments? I spent a little longer in the kitchen those days while I made the Jell-O or got ice for his water, and sometimes whispered to the Heavens, "Yes, you can take him now."

Of course, if Jack had died alone, I would have admonished myself for failing him and would have felt the shame shimmer like sweat whenever someone asked, "Where were you when he breathed his last?" I was a bad wife, I hid, and I was a good wife who knew he deserved better. The good wife stayed by his side and struggled. And prayed.

The truth is, I did nothing. The melanoma diagnosis came from a biopsy of a mole removed for cosmetic reasons, and not a medical red flag. A mole right in the middle of his sternum, the one that my five-five frame saw right there in front of my face whenever we hugged, showered together, made love, dressed, and undressed. I never examined it closely. I never prodded him to see a doctor after he remarked that it bothered him and wanted it removed. I did nothing.

The truth is, I was terrified. I wore the good-wife persona like a golden badge for all to see. I wore a mask of competence and courage for neighbors and friends. In my mirror, though, I saw panic: *I don't have a fuckin' clue what I am doing, what to expect, or how to comfort the man I love.*

I stood with Jack once the cancer was found. I squeezed time out from my workday, rearranged my hours, and rushed out for his appointments: blood tests, scans, treatments, and the dreaded results. At home, on the extension phone, I listened to updates from doctors and asked the questions Jack avoided. If Jack bucked against the information *I needed*, I asked him to step away and let the doctor talk to me. He always stayed, but I saw a tightening around his jaw and a deepened furrow on his brow, hearing the answers he didn't want to know. I took notes, even taped appointments, later transcribed, and kept the notebook of appointment summaries, test results, maps to clinics, the calendar, and any handouts the doctors or nurses gave. The first page was for questions that arose between appointments. All in my handwriting. The notebook was mine to carry. I needed a slice of order. Well-marked alphabetical tabs amidst the chaos.

I cheered each small triumph and attempted to bolster his hopes on the emotional roller coaster. We rode up with treatment, paused at the top with remission, and crashed down the other side with relapse.

This surgery got everything they could see. *Rah!*

No new tumors on the MRI this time. *Rah!*

The CT scan shows that the ones by the kidneys stayed the same size. *Rah!*

But the day came when cancer could no longer be corralled and freely roamed his body. All treatment options, even experimental ones, were exhausted. While he slept or watched television, I spent time on the computer researching treatment centers at major cancer hospitals and university medical schools. We missed cut-off dates for applications, studies were full, or we were denied because Jack had had interferon and chemo already, which might impact their trials. Doors slammed shut with, "Not accepting Stage Four patients." I yelled at the screen, "*Please, someone help him.*" Jack's oncologist checked, too. None of his colleagues at local clinics and hospitals had anything new for melanoma patients. We held no hope.

The truth is, I gave up. I lost hold of the *you-will-be-cured* torch and let it drop and extinguish like a spent match. It had grown too heavy, held aloft for too long. I quit believing Jack would beat it before he did. Many times, my spirit wanted to shout, "*Fine! You win, Cancer. Take him, but do it quickly and painlessly.*" Defeated, the bitterness soured my outlook and clanged in my ears. *Quitter.* What kind of wife was I to watch this and not fight back?

I once caught Jack as he stood half-dressed after a shower before the large rectangular bathroom mirror. He had such fine features: a hairy barrel chest, well-defined muscles on his legs and arms, chiseled cheekbones and jawline, and a few strands of reddish-blond hair from his Scottish genes among the silver. He wasn't flexing biceps or pecs like a bodybuilder. He was using his fingers to follow the path of the first two surgeries: a six-inch scar across his sternum and a smaller scar in his armpit from lymph node removal. Later, there would be a third one: an eight-incher on his back for the removal of tumors in the lung, but he wouldn't see that one without the help of a handheld mirror. Regardless, two were two too many. I backed up into the bedroom, coughed, and said, "Are you in the bathroom, Jack?" to let him know I was coming in.

This was a room we redesigned, tore down to the studs, and rebuilt in our own style: bigger shower, smaller bathtub, new tiling, white sinks, tub, and toilet, and we removed the ghastly, awful dark browns. The only benefit of the brown toilet was that one never knew if it needed cleaning. The toilet-cleaning task was on Jack's job list, and we joked that he could skip it without notice. The mirror was the only original fixture in the room.

From behind him, I wrapped my arms around Jack and leaned my face against his warm back. His moist skin held a sweet newborn's scent, soft and snuggly. I placed my hand on the mole's former spot and whispered, "I love you just the way you are." I turned him around to see his eyes brimming with tears. "You are still the most handsome man I know." A long kiss tasting of salty tears.

We stepped back; both wiped our eyes. Jack asked, "Want a smile?" He lifted his bent arms so that his elbows were above his shoulders. When his elbows were by his side, the outer edges of the scar line curved downward into a frown. With elbows raised, it stretched them upward into a smile. I forced a chuckle. But the truth was, I hated the scars, too.

Deep in the new mirror, the one that cancer handed me, far, far in the back, festering, was the stored reenactment of Jack's final morning. I turned my eyes away from the glass many times, not wanting to relive it again. But even with closed eyes, the mirror kept the vision in front of me. In this game of hide-and-seek, the demon of that final morning had found me.

The truth was, I left Jack alone when he needed me.

In our bedroom that morning, the fan rotated the warm summer air of late morning and sent wave-like ripples across the teal sheets. The blanket had long ago been folded down to the edge of the bed. The drawn blinds allowed only a few inches of the western sky's light into the room. Jack lay on his left side, his right shoulder and arm exposed; his pink head, hairless after the radiation treatment for the brain tumors a month ago, was sunken into the pillow. Jack gave off a small puff of exhaled air, his acknowledgment of my presence, as I bent down and kissed his head.

"I'm back, Bud."

Before lights out the night before, Jack's last words to me were a weak "Night," followed by a pause, and then, "Love." In the morning, he had said nothing except soft "Yeah" replies to my few questions. His silence gave me a new medical update: more of him was gone.

The hospice nurse arrived, and I escorted her upstairs to the bedroom. She was concerned that Jack had not had his morning dose of morphine. His groans whenever he was touched were an obvious sign of untreated pain. I told her that he just kept spitting out the pill that I laid on his tongue. He moved it to the edge of his tongue and used his teeth to slip it off onto the pillow. I tried three times. Each time he spat it out, I picked up the saliva-soaked pill and put it back into his mouth.

Focused on pain relief, she announced that she would give the morphine anally. Jack was trapped: he would take his morphine, and it would be against his will. I felt his resistance like a small shift in the temperature, a quiet rumble of defiance rising from his body under the sheets. I knew him, and I knew he didn't want the morphine. *I knew it.* Did he sense it was his last morning, and did he want to be as present as he could be for the final moments? That's how I would want it: to smell the roses in the vase on the nightstand, hear the robin and sparrow songs outside the window, and feel kisses on my forehead while my hand was stroked. It was how I would want it for him.

But he didn't get that because I, his caregiver, gatekeeper, and wife, ran away. My resolve and inner strength cracked when he needed me most. I intentionally left the room at a crucial moment when he needed me to be his voice. I left him to fight for himself. I left the room on the pretense of getting Jack some ice water from downstairs. I left him.

Jack's friend, the one who'd stopped by that morning for respite, helped the hospice nurse turn him on his side. The friend held him, keeping him from tipping onto his back while the nurse prepared the morphine. That was what I saw over my shoulder when I was down three stairs toward the kitchen.

It should have been me, not his friend, holding him. Maybe my hands on his back and my voice in his ear would have soothed his fears. At the very least, I should have bolted back upstairs when I heard his pleas, "No! No!" from the baby monitor in the kitchen. I should have stopped it. His final words should have been loving, quiet, peaceful, not fighting a medicine he didn't want, a medicine I knew he opposed. His final act of strength should not have been a fight against a suppository. It should have been to squeeze my hand one more time.

His cry, "No! No!" reverberated off the walls, up and down the staircase, and pounded into my chest. In the kitchen, I melted onto the floor and sobbed, "I am so sorry, Jack, I'm so sorry."

My therapist set up what is called "an empty chair" scenario in my session. I was to tell an imaginary Jack, in that empty chair, about his last morning.

"What would Jack say if he knew all this?"

Her eyes implored me to dive deeper. I caught my breath between "Oh, God, what have I done?" and "I failed him," and tried to imagine those grey-blue eyes pleading for me to find peace.

"He would roll his arms around me, pull me into his chest, and let me cry. He would listen as I apologized over and over." I imagined a kiss on my head. "He would say, '*You did your best. In those final weeks, whenever you left the bedroom and the house, you said, 'I will always love you.' And I will always love you. It was good enough, Tally, it really was.*'"

The truth is, I knew him well, and those would be his words. He would not want me to endure any further suffering. I would want that same peace for him.

With that understanding, shame's mirror cracked into shards.

Chapter 10
Silence: The First Trip Alone

It was my first cry of the morning, and I was yelling through tears. "This is your job, Jack! It's your job!"

My luggage sat open on the bed. Only one more item to pack: the pint-sized tan stuffed bear we bought early in our marriage, which was always stowed in travel bags. Whoever stayed home secretly burrowed "Fergus" in the traveler's folded shirts, or tucked him in a pocket of dress pants or inside a running shoe. No matter where I traveled, Fergus would be hidden somewhere.

A wave of loss rippled across me. Along with the sleeveless shirts, capris, and running gear I'd packed for the warm southwest days of Buckeye, Arizona, I would carry a three-piece suit of resentment, sadness, and guilt. This trip was burdensome, and I hadn't even heaved my bag down the stairs yet.

My reply to the invitation, "Yes, I'd love to visit," seemed insane now. How did I forget the details of traveling? I forgot all the ways Jack made it easier: he locked the doors and windows, toted our luggage to the car, procured extra cash just in case, let the neighbors know of our plans, helped with cleaning so that we would come back to a neat house, and stood by as my "go-fer" when this or that was needed.

My body had a childlike yearning to run out of our bedroom, open the front door, and magically be in Arizona, skipping over everything that must happen in between. My mind begged to return to the bed, to get lost in the stillness that takes no energy or thought. I wanted the "To Do" list, the checking off, the rechecking, to be turned off like a radio.

I wanted the darkness under the quilt to absorb all the sounds and thoughts that came with grief.

The bed was made, an old habit from my single days, done immediately after rising. Early in our marriage, I rose and left for work before Jack did. Bed-making was left to him, a chore often skipped, to my displeasure. When cancer began to sleep with us, the bed was never made; only sheets were changed. My old routine returned once half the bed was unused.

From the edge of the bed, I reached out and smoothed the cream-colored bedspread on his side, the right side. I imagined his atrophied limbs, nothing more than thin poles, under the linens. Ah, to feel him again, still there. Dying, but still there. My hands craved the touch. I held him so many times in this bed, Jack on his back and I on my side, my arm draped across his hairy chest, feeling his breath enter and leave his body, feeling his life, our lives. His hand would come up and hold my arm down, as if pulling me into him, deeply and securely connected.

Near the end of his life, Jack observed, "I feel like I am melting."

No, I wanted to correct him, *it's more like you left chunks of your body on operating room tables. Your blood seeped onto gauze and out through the drain tubes. I cleaned you and those tubes, tossed bandages, and every day, there was less of you than before.* But Jack said, "melting," a metaphor for dying. So late in our lives together, I viewed him differently. Was he a poet? Had I missed other moments when his words showed such depth and awareness?

Jack's energy was dissolving too. His frequent naps left me increasingly alone. Until—*when had this started?*—he was bedbound, rarely getting up except to use the bathroom. Atrophy made it difficult for him to sit upright in bed. Once on his feet, he lacked balance and required my help to make the fifteen feet to the bathroom.

In the final weeks, Jack often woke asking, "What time is it?" He, too, noticed as his naps stretched longer and longer, until he was asking instead, "What day is it?"

Yes, my love, you were melting. Slowly. Sadly. Completely.

On the pre-flight morning, dawn crept through the window and grew from a sliver on the wall to a square on the floor. I watched dust particles appear, as if they were swimming under a spotlight. The furnace kicked in, reminding me to turn it down before leaving. Another of Jack's jobs suddenly moved to my check-off list.

I held my hand over his side of the bed. I tried to imagine a pool of discarded human cells left behind from his pores, his breath. I imagined I could scoop up these cells and, like clay, add water to reconstruct his body. I wanted to feel the tingling of clasped hands, fingers tracing the contours of lips, the teasing kisses on the neck. For all those times our bodies touched, I thought my synapses must be capable of firing a memory to let me physically feel, really feel, the sensation of being held again. But under my hand, there was nothing. Nothing but a flattened blanket and an undented pillow on his side of the bed.

I flicked a glance at the digital clock on my nightstand. I had to go, and Fergus was still waiting to be packed. *Do I pack him or stop the ritual?* If I didn't pack Fergus, it would be one more way that I erased a part of us. Like the day I ran out of our checks, "Tally and Jack Reynolds," and ordered new ones in my name only. Same for address labels. *Save or toss? Now or later?* I eventually tossed the old labels and checks into the wood stove at the cabin. A part of our life together turned to ashes.

If I put a stop to our playful rituals, beginning with Fergus, what would be left? Too much changed too quickly as it was. Rising off the bed, I grabbed Fergus off the shelf, gave him a hug, and packed him under some T-shirts in my luggage.

After landing at the Phoenix airport, my travel companion called home to check in with her husband, get updates on their children, and chat about the trip. My house was empty; no one was waiting for the details of my flight. Only the dog sitter knew of my departure and return. I missed calling home. And later that day, I had no one to call to tell the story of how I found a bear hidden in my suitcase.

Within Jack, there was an imaginative little boy with an adolescent sense of comedy. I loved that boyish side of him. When he traveled with Fergus, he gave the bear a goofy, animated voice. The calls always made me chuckle.

"Mom, Mom!" Jack would say in a high-pitched voice. "I'm here with Jack! It was a bumpy plane ride, and I thought I would get sick. But I didn't."

I would feign surprise. "You little rascal, Fergus, did you sneak off again?"

"Mom, I had to go. It's my job."

"Okay," I would concede. "Don't you get into trouble. Just be sure you two come home safe."

Fergus' voice was silent, too, on the day Jack died.

Chapter 11
The Bed: Memories Around Our Bed

How much easier it would have been if Jack hadn't died in our bed. If only he had died in a private hospice room, or in the small New York hotel where we had our last birthday adventure together, a mere six weeks before his passing. If only the hospital bed ordered had arrived a month or two earlier, instead of four hours before his last breath. If only, once his body was removed, someone else would have stripped the bed, cleaned the linens, sanitized the mattress and the bed frame, and provided fresh sheets for the next occupant. Another bed would have been simpler, kinder.

After phoning the hospice office to inform them of Jack's death, a task I was told was most urgent and needed to be timely, the next calls were to my mother, my little sister in Texas, my older brother in Arizona, and the first person at the top of a phone tree of friends. My last call was to Glenda. My fingers trembled dialing the phone as I felt the slow disintegration of my mind. I was pushing to function through a vast darkness with only a burning match to light my way. I dreaded repeating the story, hearing myself speak the same words again and again as if I were a parrot and not a loving wife. It was hard to comprehend that Glenda and I had talked on the phone just yesterday when Jack was still alive.

"It's bad, Glenda," I explained. "He's stopped eating. A couple of ice chips, that's all the fluid he's getting. He still gets up to use the bathroom, but it's painful for him to stand and walk."

"I'm so sorry, Tally. I remember how it was with my stepfather in those last weeks. It's just awful." Silence grew between us.

"Call me," she finally said. "Call me the second things change. You understand?"

I nodded while facing the kitchen wall.

Now Glenda arrived, less than an hour after I relayed the news. She came straight from a visit to her mother, who lived in a neighboring town and was beginning to show signs of dementia. Glenda knocked softly, knowing better than to ring that jarring doorbell. Opening the door, I was pulled into a hug. Glenda's floral-scented hair pressed against my cheek, and the cool of the car's air conditioner radiated from her shirt. I knew I needed help from this levelheaded woman.

Glenda was like me in so many ways: both of us were junior high school counselors, and we had the same body type. My hair was darker, short, and straight, while hers was auburn and naturally curly, but we'd joked that I was a twin sister her mother forgot to tell her about.

I led Glenda up the stairs. In the bedroom, with her arm across my shoulders, we stood before the bed with Jack lying on his left side. We said little until the memorial-home personnel arrived. A fan rotated the warm summer air around us.

One of us went downstairs when we heard the knock. One of us opened the front door, explained the situation, and showed the men upstairs. One of us stayed in the room. These steps are a blur, but suddenly there were two middle-aged men standing with us in the bedroom.

They were here for Jack's remains. *Remains?* That's what the hospice nurse called Jack, too, when I called. I winced. What a sterile word to denote his body, his physical temple, the heart, muscles, and sagging skin of an almost six-foot man that held that kind spirit.

Both men had average builds and nondescript auras. They were not husky football players, which I had expected for this occupation. One had dark hair, and both wore white polos and khakis. I trusted they were capable and well-trained. One said, "We are not in a hurry. You tell us when." Both stood against the wall to wait, eyes downcast and hands folded in front of them as if in silent prayer.

Immediately after his last heartbeat, I had slipped behind Jack on the bed to hug him one last time. I whispered, "I will always love you," into his ear. I took off his wedding ring. And now these men were in our room.

"Take all the linen with you," I barked at them suddenly. "All of it."

It was unlike me not to say *please* or *thank you,* but I never wanted to see those colors again. Death and teal were now coupled. I kissed Jack's head one more time, and, nodding to the men, I left the room. I'd seen enough. I went out of the bedroom door and down the stairs, past the main floor, down past the landing with its access to the garage, and down a few more steps toward the cool daylight basement. From there, I'd hear their descent but didn't see the remains sway, as if in a summer hammock, out the door.

From my perch on the stairs, I had a clear view of the basement: the television and two-seater sofa with autumn-colored plaid upholstery, which we detested but deemed "good enough" for its bargain price. Closing my eyes, I imagined Jack with a head of silver-red-blond hair, thinning on top, wearing a T-shirt from a wrestling tournament he officiated, hairy legs showing underneath his shorts, socked feet on the flip-up footrest. His glasses, with round tortoiseshell frames, reflected the light from the TV. Watching a game, a history documentary, or "How Do They Build That?" Sound down low. I imagined him snoring.

Glenda kept an eye on the men upstairs while I imagined it all. Someone must have pulled the blanket and bedspread off. A hand gently on Jack's shoulder, another on his hip, one man must have rolled Jack from his side onto his back. Together, they must have pulled the fitted sheet off the corners of the mattress to create the sling. Perhaps they tucked the pillowcases around him like cushions, and then covered him with the flat sheet in preparation to take him down the flight of stairs to the car.

In the basement, my heart screamed, *Kiss him one last time!* I yelled up the stairs, "Wait, wait, wait!" and dashed up to find the men just four steps out of the bedroom. "I need to kiss him goodbye." The man at the head gently and easily unwrapped the sheet to expose Jack's head. I was not the first to make this final request, I thought: these men were ready for last-minute pleas. A final kiss on a cool head. I returned to the basement.

"They're leaving," Glenda called from the landing moments later.

I unfolded myself, scurried to the front door, and stood on the stoop with her. I expected a black hearse, but a gold Honda SUV was parked in the driveway. I was stunned. Where did they place this almost six-foot man? In the back with the middle seats folded down? Tucked across the middle as if he were three passengers long?

I waved to the gold car as it drove my husband away and whispered, "Bye, Jack." I had yet to cry. After I closed the front door, we stood in the entry.

"I can stay longer," Glenda offered.

"No." Shock stilled the air around and within me.

She hugged me until I let go. Placing her hands on my shoulders, Glenda looked hard into my eyes. "Call me, you understand, if you need anything. I don't care how late. Do you hear me?"

With a small nod and a voice that came from somewhere far away, I said, "Thanks for everything, Glenda." I locked the door behind her, already mindful of my safety. This moment was the beginning of being truly alone, the moment I had been practicing for weeks while Jack slept.

I walked back up to the bedroom in slow plods, dreamlike, feeling as if the stairs went on and on, as if I might never reach the top. But I did get there, stopping at our open bedroom door to look at the bed: Glenda had remade it with the cream-colored sheets.

Annie B was curled up against Jack's pillow.

The dam broke. I knelt on the ground, rocked, and wept.

I asked the men to take all the teal linens, and I saw Jack carrying them out. But somehow, one teal pillowcase stayed behind, the one he lay his head on those last days. I found it in the basement laundry room and pulled it to my face to inhale his smell, his sweet, earthly smell, something between red licorice and newly dug-up soil. I brought it back to the bedroom, unwashed, and tucked it under the pillow on Jack's side. Each night before turning off the light, I pulled it out, hugged it to my chest with a deep inhale, and returned it underneath. *I miss you so much.*

It's interesting how couples develop bed-related routines. On our travels, in various hotels, in the guest rooms of friends, we always slept on the same sides of the bed. On a few rare occasions, when one of us flopped down for a quick nap on the wrong side, it felt odd. Invariably, we switched back before the lights went out. Without Jack, I would sleep on my usual left side of the bed and let Annie B stretch out on Jack's side.

During the last six weeks of his life, I became accustomed to seeing him sleeping on his side whenever I came into the room. After he passed, I often walked upstairs to tell him something. When I used the bathroom or put laundry away, I wanted him in the bed, still here with me. In the middle of the night, I reached for him, always surprised that the bed was empty.

A year later, I put the house up for sale and laid Annie B to rest. The real estate agent requested staging the master bedroom with a fancier bed. I recognized this as the right time to act, time for a new bed, a symbol of letting go. Janet helped me remove the old mattress. Janet and her twin sister, Deborah, often did dog care for Annie B when Jack and I traveled or got stuck at school. Janet and I grunted as we slid the mattress on its side down the stairs, stood it upright for turns at the landing, and took it out the front door to hoist and tie it onto Jack's truck. We drove in silence to the dump. As Janet untied the ropes, I kissed the mattress. "Goodbye, Jackson," and then, to the bed, "Thanks for all the memories."

I called out to Janet, "Ready to toss? On three. One, two, three," before we heaved the mattress off the truck into the large dumpster, amidst construction debris, yard waste, and broken children's toys.

That same day, I dismantled the bedframe and passed it along to a young couple in need of a bed. Parts and pieces of our lives would be unbolted and carried to the truck, removed from the house, just like that.

I slept, for a time, in the guest room bed in the basement. When I turned off the light, it was strange to be in the darkness. Jack's light wasn't on, and I didn't hear the crinkling of book pages being turned, or his negotiation: "Just a few more." At my request, he finally turned off his light, kissed me goodnight, and spooned me for a few minutes until we both rolled back onto our own sides.

Eventually, when I sold the house and found a new one, I encased Jack's pillowcase in plastic bags for the move, but his scent was gone when I unpacked the linen box. Another loss.

In the "mistress bedroom" of my new house, I slept on our old guest bed for months until I found a new frame, cherry wood with a metal *fleur-de-lis* pattern on the foot and headboards. A new mattress, too. I tried the middle of the mattress as my "sleeping spot," but the abundance of space reminded me of the emptiness. I returned to the left side.

When I adopted a Rat Terrier old-age rescue, nine months after moving in, I did everything I could to make Anna comfortable in her new home. Our first night together, I placed her on the bed and watched her stretch out on my left side.

"Oh, little Anna, that's my spot." But I couldn't disturb her. I slid into Jack's right side for the first time.

Chapter 12
[Poem]

Bed

After donating our bed

the last task was heaving

the queen mattress into

the dumpster. Before releasing

my grip, I kissed it, letting go

of what was shared. Dreams,

whispers, silence, distance,

apologies,

holding, kisses,

lovemaking,

plans, gratitude,

regrets, pecks "Goodnight,'

after work naps,

viruses, infections, surgeries,

disease, new

house, new walls, coming home

late or too sick or snoring,

in the cold bed downstairs,

sleeping alone, a new puppy taking up

more of the bed than anticipated.

Comfort of "our bed" after travel, too

much sleep, not enough,

nightmares, one early riser,

making pancakes, back to bed,

with morning papers, alarms

not going off, dashing

out. Sleeping in on snow days,

no-school mornings, changing

the sheets. Middle of the night

peeks at each other.

Birthdays, anniversaries,

love cards left

on pillows.

Shared tears, fears, and hopes,

"Is he still breathing?"

all his for comfort, not sleeping

with him,

an inflatable twin on the floor,

an unused hospital bed

This is the bed he died in.

Not sleeping

Not sleeping

Not sleeping

Sleeping only on my side

of the bed. Looking for him

on his side. Imagining him

there, fading memories, and

still teary,

Not sleeping well

New smaller house and new, smaller dog

Different frame and mattress

Still not sleeping

Chapter 13
Time: Hours and Days Slip Away

What can I say about time as a widow? Like those sci-fi novels with time warps and parallel universes, I held my own time fantasy. I wanted to travel back fifteen years before cancer came into our lives, slow down the clock, and the turns of calendar pages. As a visitor to our past, I would relive minor conflicts with patience. I would prevent the long silences that followed harsh words and make quicker apologies. We would walk hand-in-hand more. Have more adventures. More tenderness.

But when cancer was consuming Jack's body and his pain was excruciating, and I felt his grunts and groans twisting my own intestines, my fantasies went in the other direction. *Run, Clock, run. Race faster to the end line.*

Time was an elusive enemy. A hell. It was also an ally.

The time between "Jack is alive" and "Jack is dead" was paper-thin, immeasurable. In that sliver of a second, I was left the sole possessor of our past: "I *was* his wife. He *was* my husband." I tasted bitterness in my mouth whenever I spoke of past and present in the same sentence: "Jack and I loved shopping at Costco together. I detest going alone now." I yearned to spit phrases like *he's gone, he passed,* and *he died* into the ground and stomp on them wildly.

While grocery shopping or walking Annie B in the neighborhood, conversations with neighbors and friends inevitably circled around to, "What are you doing with yourself?" I heard an unspoken ellipsis at the end of the question: "...now that Jack is dead."

Do I tell them about standing in the garage before Jack's truck and tools, with the smell of freshly cut pine wood, newly mixed cement, or the hot solder of copper pipes whirling around me? Do I speak of the drive to the homeless shelter where I donated his warm jackets before the winter cold, hugged and kissed each article goodbye? What about his final meals in the refrigerator that I can neither eat nor toss? How I knelt regularly before the CD player, listening to Josh Groban's "To Where You Are" on repeat? How, after hearing some gossipy tidbit in the cul-de-sac, I wanted to race upstairs to him in *our* bed: "Ya gotta hear this, Bubba. Linda just told me…"

Visitors came into the house, their eyebrows raised as I began to reminisce: "Jack and I put in those walls and added speakers. It was quite a feat." Or, "We bought that iris watercolor print. Such a funny story." But I don't give the details, and they don't ask. *When will she let him go?*

Time ran amok, jumbled words and thoughts between past, present, past, present, tossed around like bingo balls in the cage. I never knew which verb tense would pop out from my lips. Either one felt wrong and poorly timed.

Sitting on a kitchen stool one morning, I watched the dawn light peek over the neighbor's roof, sending sunbeams through my window. With cold cereal and hot tea before me, Annie B curled up on her bed a few feet away, my mind skittered out an odd thought: I wish I owned a tall oak grandfather clock, something loud to denote time's passage.

My analog watch, with a howling wolf on its face, gold trim, and a worn brown leather band, was shelved with unused jewelry. I stopped wearing it the first summer after retirement. Time drove my weekdays for thirty-one years, with classes, appointments, and meetings. Often, lunches involved quick bites of fruit between visits with adults or students, or a sandwich chewed quietly while on the phone. I once joked with a colleague that I could shake enough crumbs from my keyboard to have a midafternoon snack. As a new retiree, I was ready to float through my days without the pressure to fit more than humanly possible into each hour. Gloriously, I silenced the alarm clock and let my body tell me when to rise.

Cancer came back five months into retirement. Jack's medical appointments dictated where and when we had to be, so I retrieved the watch from the shelf. I sighed: the second hand was still; the battery was dead. After replacing the battery, I wore it until Jack's final day. Two months later, again, I lifted the watch from its place and found the battery dead again. Time stood still.

But a grandfather clock, with a large glass face, black hands, dots of painted gold, and scallops of wood trim, standing majestically in the entry of the house, would remind me that I endured the passing of time without Jack. The sashay of the pendulum would swing seconds back and forth in sync with my own heartbeats, with a soft "*tick...tick...tick*". The chimes would bounce off the walls, up and down the stairs, and into the corners of these empty rooms, and announce that I survived another hour. Twelve strikes marked half a day's passage.

But that isn't how time passed with Jack gone. Instead, the house clocks ran slower and slower. The hours dragged the minutes behind them like stubborn children resisting a bath. The second hand peeked out from behind the others shyly, and occasionally, I swear, stopped entirely. I lived in this slow-moving world between his death and my life alone. My sluggish legs mimicked a tamed elephant, one slow bend of the knee and methodical step at a time. Over and over, until I reached the bathroom. Or kitchen. Or back to our bed. Slow, sad strides. Healing measured by the time that passed between my bouts of crying, balled up on the floor.

Grieving was easier in the light of day when I sat at the kitchen table, trying to read the morning news. Comics were the easiest: short snippets of humor, digestible without deep thought. The windows let in the colors of the surrounding maples, alders, and evergreens. The room seemed bigger with natural light. But when the darkness stalked in from behind those trees, the walls moved in too. So did the walls of my mind, pressed inward by cold silence. Another day gone, without any distinction from yesterday. Like grasping at smoke, I had nothing to distinguish one twenty-four hours from another.

The numbers of the digital clock seemed to nod off in the star-filled night, slowing the passage of hours. After lying in bed for what felt like four or five hours, I opened my eyes and assumed dawn was nearing. But when I checked the clock, only twenty minutes had passed. I turned away again, avoiding the clock, but the blue numbers drew me back. Only another fifteen minutes had gone by. More time to face the empty side of the bed in the dark.

In the pre-dawn light, in bed with Annie B nestled next to my hip, I woke again and stretched my limbs under the covers. *What do I have to get done today?* Today I wanted to prove I wasn't wasting time. I wanted to cross off something, *anything*, from the ever-growing "to-do" list. I pulled out fresh underwear from the drawer and dressed in yesterday's bra, shorts, t-shirt left on top of the dresser, and grabbed a sweatshirt for the morning chill. After Annie B's meal, we would make our way down the porch stairs to the cul-de-sac for her "duties."

At the kitchen counter, I ate a slice of toast and made a cup of Earl Grey before I moved to the dining room to begin the workday. At the dining table, I opened a folder, then realized I wanted another sip of hot tea. I tossed the folder back on the table and retrieved my cup from the counter. While in the kitchen, I noticed an item from yesterday's mail that needed filing. Upstairs to the study's file cabinet, but instead of filing, I tossed the envelope on the floor in front of the cabinet with all the other unfiled items. Turning, I spied an unopened utility bill on the desk. I sat down, opened the envelope, read the amount owed, and knew I should bring it to the bill bin downstairs in the kitchen so I wouldn't lose it for the first-of-the-month bill-paying day. But first, I checked my email. I opened my inbox, browsed through messages from friends, deleted spam, and typed out a few lines for a blog entry. Annie B trotted into the study.

"Do you need to go outside?"

Annie B telegraphed with her ears forward and a slight head tilt: *Sure do.*

I rose from my desk without shutting down the computer and headed outside for our walk. My tea had gone cold.

The silver metal clock on the kitchen wall signaled that it should be dinnertime. I didn't remember lunch. No twelve strikes of a grandfather clock as a reminder. The only meals I prepared consistently were Annie B's. With her internal timer, she sought me out and stood where I could not step forward without tripping into her diminishing fifty pounds. Teetering on those old hips, unable to sit without straining to get back up, she gave me her hungry look: her black ears flattened to her head, her tail drooped to the floor, and her brown-turning-blue eyes pleading.

"Are you hungry?" I teased. Annie B's ears snapped forward, and her tail gave a slow wave, as if to say, *You're late.*

"I'm sorry, I'm late."

I heard myself say this so often that I began to worry about early-onset dementia. I set alarm clocks for morning appointments, but forgot to press the "on" button. Or worse, I didn't set the alarm to "a.m.," so it sounded in the "p.m." Even when I rose on time and proceeded with my morning routine, somehow the clock scampered out ahead of me. I lived like the White Rabbit to the Queen's tea party: *I'm late, I'm late, I'm late.*

There were Post-it notes on mirrors and doors for items that I needed to take with me when I left the house. Some were placed by the door to the garage, where I thought *I couldn't possibly miss seeing this when I step out.* But "I'm sorry, I left it at home" became the verbal bookend to "I'm sorry, I'm late."

"I want my life back the way it was!"

My scream startled poor Annie B from her late afternoon nap. My fists shook at the ceiling. My face flushed with fury, triggered by one too many small pains and disasters from the week. In my hand was yet another bill addressed to both of us. *He's not here,* I yelled at it. Yesterday, an envelope I'd mailed was returned, undelivered because I forgot the stamp. Another day, the mail was returned because I forgot to write one of the four numbers of the street address. I wanted all the folders and boxes off the dining room table. I wanted to create a dam of paper behind my arm as I swept down the table's length, to cheer as it all flew off the end. All that would remain on the dining room table would be today's newspaper, a gardening catalog, a personal letter or two, and my teacup.

I wanted to be outside weeding, taking off dead blossoms, and trimming back branches. Or amidst the trees in the back, on the deck that we built, working on a Sudoku. I wanted to slide into memories while the aroma of chocolate chip walnut cookies filled the kitchen, and watch Jack sneak a handful off the cooling rack. I'd like to curl up on the couch downstairs next to him, hold his hand, and watch a

Mariners baseball game. I wanted his help with the chores. I wanted to feel rested, unhurried.

More and more, I wanted back a live, healthy Jack. I wanted to reverse time, a crazy thought that only made me angrier. I felt locked in a two-year-old's tantrum. As a counselor, I knew that behind the emotion of anger was fear. Anger was easier to express; fear meant admitting weakness. I feared I would never come out of this grief.

Will every minute of every hour of the rest of my life be tinted with sadness? Will I die alone?

I heard Annie B's groan and realized I'd folded into a ball, sobbing. She shuffled toward me, disliking it when her human cried, and came to lick away the tears. I caught my breath, wiped my face with my sleeve, and circled my arm around her shoulders. "We'll make it through this hell, Girl, we will." Her tail gave a slow wag of agreement.

My mind was once neat and orderly, like the closet of a compulsive organizer. As a school counselor, I once organized and executed an entire week's worth of required state testing for my building. Three grades with three different tests at three different lengths. Today, everything in my home is in utter shambles. Stacks are ransacked, shelf contents are scattered, and clothing items once sorted by color and style are teetering off hangers, if hung at all. I can't borrow library books or tools from friends; I am unable to return them in a timely fashion.

Widowed Brain.

One day, my only task was to write two checks. Two checks. That's all. After breakfast in the kitchen, I went up the fourteen stairs to my study and grabbed the checkbook from the desk. I held the navy-blue checkbook in my hand, even checked to see that the pen was still stored inside. Back down the same fourteen stairs, I walked the six steps to the dining room table and sat down in front of the bills I needed to pay.

But had I arrived at the table without the checkbook? Poof! It was gone. I stood before the table, trying to understand where I could have possibly stopped between there and here. Blank. I remembered the widower in my support group who once found his hammer in the freezer. I checked the freezer: not there.

After an hour of rummaging for the checkbook, I was crying, pleading from the floor of Jack's closet.

I want my husband and my brain back, God. Please?

Every clock in the house seemed to taunt me. *And what did you do today?*

On my life timeline, there was a great demarcation: there was *the before,* and *the afterward,* my own personal version of B.C. ("Before Chaos") and A.D. ("After Death"). Like a countdown in reverse, I was constantly adding up the time that came after June 28, 2008, 12:52 p.m.

"Twenty minutes ago, Jack passed."

"He's been gone twenty-five hours."

"Two weeks and three days."

"Tomorrow will be four months."

A few friends asked, "How long ago did Jack die?"

Sometimes I found a place in the conversation to toss it in: "Fourteen months already." Other times, when asked, I bit my tongue and pretended to do the math. But I knew. To the minute.

Eventually, time shifted and blurred so that I no longer mentally computed the exact weeks and days at a moment's notice. How long has it been since Jack died? Time played with the math.

"Two years and a couple of months."

"About twenty-nine months."

"Still feels like yesterday."

Gradually, I accepted the truth that time offers. Jack became my late husband, and time does not stand still.

Chapter 14
One: Selling Our House and His Coffee Mug

Whenever I opened the kitchen cabinet, up there on the top shelf, I saw his Sunday ceramic mug, the half of a matching pair. I treated it like an artifact in a museum. Occasionally I brought it down, secured it in both hands, and felt the cool porcelain in my palms. When I hooked my index finger into the handle and wrapped my thumb around the cup, I imagined his hand still there: the warmth of his skin, the rough calluses, the hairy knuckles.

This was enough to overwhelm me, grief buckling my knees, the mug snuggled against my chest as I sobbed and rocked on the wood floor. When the tears eventually ebbed, they always did, my breathing came in sighs, and I stood.

That simple mug held so much. The original pair was a holiday gift from a neighbor who knew us well. In the soft tan background of each cup, small black paw prints walked around the words "DOG LOVER." The rim was low enough to fit under the drip of the home espresso machine, yet wide enough to hold a twelve-ounce drink. The neighbor moved away, and Jack was gone, but the empty Sunday mugs remained with me.

For Jack and me, Sunday unfolded like the newspaper laid out in sections, casually perused and slowly turned. Sundays were oblivious to the workday's demands. Sunday sauntered in like Annie B, no longer rushing after squirrels or strangers. "Take it slow like me," her eyes told us.

Dog care, breakfast, and breakfast dishes were the sole morning activities, culminating with what I called "dessert": a hot mocha and the entire Sunday paper devoured before noon. Starting with the comics, I moved through every section, including the ads, while Jack focused on sports and local news.

We were patient with each other's interruptions.

"Can you believe what this legislator has proposed?"

"You gotta read what 'Dear Abby' said to this woman."

"Guess who they let go in that trade for Johnson?"

Shy of a year after Jack's passing, one cloudy Sunday morning after a light breakfast of toast and hot green tea, I took the two mugs out of the cabinet and set them down on the countertop. I played with the idea of getting the espresso machine out, but that seemed too laborious, too many steps for one drink. I peered into Jack's mug, checking for dust or dead bugs. Around the base and up one side were fine, hair-like lines. I rubbed my finger inside the mug, praying that it was just a spider's web. No, these were cracks. Not from a careless slip of the hand, not from rattling around in the dishwasher. Cracks without reason or cause.

I cared for this cracked mug because, simply, it was his. His mug, the one he held, drank from, washed along with mine, and placed on the shelf, was part of a set. But the crack also felt like a harbinger of larger things to come. I feared there were other silent breaks or failures in the house, a disaster gone unnoticed until a flip of a switch. I began to feel I was living in a house of cards. I feared the windy days and wondered, "What will fall first, and what after that, and then after that?"

I once saw a television comedy skit of a Charlie Chaplin look-alike holding a long rake, whose job was to push up a huge pile of garbage that loomed several feet above his head. As soon as he got one section stable, another began to collapse, spewing trash at his feet. He would scurry to press his tool against the weak spot, rest a moment against the pile, then dash off to another falling section, repeating the process several times around the pile. It was funny to watch this man's futile attempts to stop the avalanche of garbage.

With the responsibility of the house falling to me, it was I who scurried around trying to maintain what was falling apart. I was not laughing. My life wasn't funny.

Whenever Jack walked into a room carrying "Bertha," as we called the big sledgehammer, I knew he had on his "destruction shirt." Jack approached demolition the same way he did pruning or taking down trees: he would take it all down and deal with my cries of, "Stop! Stop! You ruined it!" later. I can still feel the flying bits of sheetrock as Bertha smashed through an unwanted wall, and wreckage ricocheted off me.

Jack took a school-quarter leave from teaching after his first bout with chemo and started the remodel of the kitchen. He lacked the stamina to work the nine-hour teaching day and needed frequent naps, but he could still swing a sledgehammer. Bertha gave him a distraction and purpose. On some level, he knew what I knew: cancer reduced the number of days left in his life. He would leave a remodeled kitchen behind, his gift for me.

Standing in the kitchen with Jack's mug in both hands, I closed my eyes. I smelled his sweat, the way it mingled with the dust in the air as he tore out the cooking island, cabinets, and countertops. I could hear the *bang* of his framing gun shooting nails into new wood, and the shrill whine of screws drilled into sheetrock. I smiled and remembered Jack, mud-splattered, as the texture gun sprayed as much on him as it did on the walls. I could see the taut tendons in his hand and arm as he wrenched the new pipes and faucet tightly. And then there was his profanity, coming out from the switches, outlets, and can-o-lights where he got zapped by a live wire after ignoring my pleas to turn off the current. We painted together, but only after I did the tedious prep work. Jack had no patience for the blue painter's tape, it stuck to his fat fingers more than the trim, and I was impatient if I found the paint had bled under the tape. The house held the content and the memories of our twenty-six years together. I could not go on living if I stayed there.

If I sold the house within two years of Jack's death, I would save up to $250,000 in capital gains payments, an IRS tax break for widows and widowers. But this meant every stage of selling a house, clearing and packing, and showing, had to occur in the cruel window between the day after death and the second death anniversary. Whoever made that law didn't understand that for those first two years, getting out of bed each morning is a widow's triumph, and donning clean clothes an act of courage.

I needed that tax break. That decision to sell was made by my internal calculator, a cold, logic-ruled part of myself that dealt with finances. Factoring in a very slow housing market, the unique floor plan of the house, and the average home in the area being on the market for a hundred days, I was jammed against a wall to act quickly. Few homes were sold in the winter season; holidays kept people where they were. In June, a few weeks before the first anniversary of Jack's death, I signed a contract to put the house on the market within months. I held the vision of a "Sold" sign dangling on the white post at the curb. It had to happen before the second anniversary.

Before the first anniversary of Jack's passing came around the bend, there were other losses. My mother's death was nine months after

Jack's. This was the loss that left me an orphan, but it was not one that left me most devastated. The distance between my mother and me did not mend with her prognosis of kidney failure. I was at peace with her passing, relieved that I no longer bolted up in bed whenever the phone rang in the late hours. But, as with some deaths in a family, fractures elsewhere in the family grew greater. In my case, those fissures that were not visible beforehand became apparent at the memorial. With my mother's passing, I also lost a sense of closeness with my little sister, Beth, whom I had once described as a best friend who happened to be family. Suddenly, this woman seemed to have little in common with me; I lost an important confidante who knew my history. Incredibly, the death of Mother and loss of Beth foreshadowed further devastation that came only ten weeks later: the agony of laying to rest our Annie B.

Annie B's fifteen-year-old hindquarters deteriorated to the point that I was carrying her fifty-pound black-and-tan body up and down the stairs. She no longer wanted to sleep with me upstairs, preferring her heated dog bed on the main floor. One day, I lifted her from her bed to carry her outside for her "duties," and she didn't nip at my hand as I scooped her up. At that point, we both knew her final day was nearing.

Annie B's brown eyes, full of love, still followed my movements whenever she heard my steps. I convinced myself that she had a few good days still left in her.

Impossible. Simply impossible to let her go.

A dog-loving friend came over. She observed Annie B for a few seconds, then said, "It's time, Tally."

"I know, I know, but we're only three weeks away from the first anniversary of Jack's passing. I need her here with me."

I felt the red shame rise into my cheekbones as my head drooped. I would never hurt an animal or ignore their pain. Keeping her alive wasn't loving or humane, but since Jack left, Annie B had filled a crucial role: another spirit, another focus in the house, other sounds besides mine. I peered into her brown eyes and finally accepted what I had been resisting.

I'm sorry, Ms. B. I know. This is my job.

I called the vet, made the appointment, telling myself, *Don't look back. Do it now before you change your mind. This is the right thing to do. This is your job.*

Two days later, I showed the vet and her technician into the house. The vet tech was a former student of mine, a small-world coincidence. Kneeling before Annie B, I averted my eyes when they gave her the first sedation shot. I held her in my arms, whispering into her ear. I thanked her for the love and laughter she gave us. I asked her to tell Jack that I missed him when she got to the Rainbow Bridge. Finally, I kissed her goodbye. Normally, she would have licked my tears from my face; instead, they fell onto her head. Annie B had her final moments cozied up in her bed in the only house she ever knew. I nodded to the vet to signify that I was ready for the second shot to stop her heart.

The house became quieter as the first anniversary approached. No more clicking of Annie B's nails on the wood floors or long sighs as she plopped into her bed. No tail thumping as I walked into the room. No crunching of kibble or lapping of water in the kitchen.

There was no one for me to greet aloud in the morning. No watching the clock for feedings. No rushing home from being out with friends to carry her out for her "duties." No bending over into her bed, kissing the top of her head, scratching behind her ears, or massaging her sore shoulders and hips.

Without Annie B, I woke each day to worry only about what I needed. Me, all me. I learned a new alone.

Contrary to agent and market predictions, the house sold in twenty-two days. I could no longer move at a leisurely pace to clean out storage spaces and organize what was left. My timeline shrank to match a real estate contract of forty-five days, out of the house by late September. I didn't have time to make slow decisions or hug the past.

One morning, tired of sorting, packing, and taping boxes, I sat on the stairs and eyed the chaos before me. Every room had opened or sealed, marked boxes, low hedges of cardboard that I walked over and around to get anywhere. I held my tired head in my hands and tasted my tears.

Oh, God, what have I done? Help me, Bud, God help me.

That evening, I sat at my desk, a glass of Malbec by my side, a plate of Havarti and apple slices for dinner. I booted up a house-finding site. With a few mouse clicks to set parameters, I perused my options.

Nope. Can't live there, with a neighbor's view of my patio.

Nope, that yard is so barren.

The room's tiny! The kitchen needs a complete gutting. No.

Reading was more difficult than I imagined. I closed my browser.

I tried again during a lunch break a couple of weeks later, with even less success. I was wasting time on the net while I should have been moving boxes into my two large, rented storage units ten miles away from the house. The cabin garage became a third storage space, but it required a four-hour round-trip drive.

And then there was the cruise. Well before the thought of selling had ever entered my mind, when Jack was still alive, I booked a ten-day East Mediterranean cruise for that October. That trip was supposed to be something special to do in the last fall of Jack's life, but instead, I would travel in his memory, ten days after closing.

Even if I found an adequate house to buy, the negotiations and closing documents could take weeks or longer. I didn't have time. The best solution was to turn off the computer, spend fall and winter at the cabin, and stay in the guest rooms of friends when I had appointments or events in town. In the spring, I'd start house shopping again.

Every single item in the house had my fingerprints on it and was marked with my decision: "Store," "Donate," or "Garbage." Sorting Jack's possessions provided me with an illusion of control. During his dying, I was adrift; all I could do was watch, wait, and pray. I wanted my world back the way it was before his death, but if I couldn't reconstruct that old life, I was at least going to regain a small sense of order in this new normal.

In packing for the move, I realized that, despite layers of bubble wrap, Jack's cracked mug would not survive the pressure of other wrapped items in a box of kitchen wares. I imagined myself crying over the mug's sharp shards as they fell onto my lap in a new, empty house. Determined to do it my way rather than leaving it to the fates, I made the decision: *Let his mug go. Now.*

The closing inspection required shoring up the large back deck we rebuilt years ago. The contractor was an eager young man of slender build. He dug deeper holes and laid forms for the eventual cement pour around the existing posts. I walked outside to look at a posthole, with Jack's mug clutched to my heart. How I wish I could experience a miracle, pull it away from my body, and see that it had been made whole by the force of my love.

I'd thought the same way with Jack: if I loved harder and prayed more, I should be able to cure him. But the prayers changed with time. When faced with the possibility of a major stroke, I prayed to God, *"Take all of him; don't leave this active, spirited man paralyzed in body and thought."* Eventually, my prayers were for a painless and quick death. The powerlessness of loving a dying man was an awful lesson: to continue to love without a miracle in sight.

Out under the deck, closing my eyes, I envisioned a Sunday morning.

We are both in our sweats and slippers, both with our bedheads, short hair rumpled but given a cursory brushing, enough to knock down cowlicks and appear dignified enough to walk the dog out in the cul-de-sac among other early risers. The batter bowl, skillet, and plates from a breakfast of pancakes are in the sink for later cleanup. I am at the table already, separating the newspaper into sections. Back in the kitchen, I can hear the gurgling of the espresso machine while Jack froths the milk, and the clinks of the spoon against the side of the mug as he stirs together the shot of espresso, milk, and flavoring.

Jack hands me my mocha with a grin. From the warm "Dog Lover" cup in my hands, I smell the espresso and chocolate in the rising steam. I smell the start of Sunday.

"Hmmm. Extra foam?" I eye the heaping mound in my mug. "Where's yours?"

"Right here." Jack presents his mug, with a skin on top. "My foam must have slipped off into yours."

"Yeah, right," I say to his sheepish look. "Got caught, didn't ya?"

"I know you love the foam," he said, defending his barista work. "And I adore you."

"As I do you."

I smile at his smile. Before sipping my drink, I pause. From my heart, I feel a warm wave of love. Clicking our mugs with a toast to our lives, I turn back to the comics. Sunday resumes.

I opened my moistened eyes and stared at the cracked mug in my sweaty palms. Under the canopy of cedar, maple, and evergreen trees, I watched the singing birds skip among the branches and inhaled the warm scent of pine mixed with stirred dirt. There was an occasional spark in the air from an insect's iridescent wings as it darted through the stripes of sunrays and disappeared back into the shadows. Mosaic tiles of light formed on the ferns, downed trees, and last fall's decaying maple leaves on the back slope. It was just me, the mug, and the house that would no longer be mine in a matter of weeks. The mug contained so much.

I miss you so much, Bud. So much it hurts to breathe.

My resolve waned as I stood there, as if the rising heat of the day was drying out something inside of me. The flashback weakened me. Maybe another time? But at another time, I would have to face this same process again, the teetering between past and present. I didn't know if I could handle that. Shaking a fist at my doubts, I quickly pulled the mug away from my chest and hurled it into the post hole. I heard it shatter.

I couldn't look down.

Cold crept up from the soil and rippled over my skin. I had removed one more thing of Jack's from this world. Who was I to hold such power? Yet a small voice within trembled out, "You did it." I faced what initially felt impossible, went through the searing pain, and finished the task. Again. Like picking up Jack's ashes in three boxes. Like finding the three separate spots for their burials. Like signing the house-selling papers. I had earned another stripe on the sleeve, or a medal of courage. I felt a poppy-seed–sized force within me, a new determination, a drive to not completely succumb to this hell of being the one left behind.

Empty-handed, with watery eyes, I stumbled along the path to the front of the house. At the porch, I pulled the edge of my tank top, wiped my eyes, and with a long sigh, entered. The one remaining DOG LOVER mug waited in the kitchen to be bubble-wrapped and placed in a box. Eventually, I would find a new home, bring my mug, a survivor itself, and place it on a shelf to greet me in the morning.

Chapter 15
Rings: What Do I Do With Them?

"Will you take off your ring someday? Or move it over to your right hand?"

I was out for coffee with a well-meaning friend. As her questions hung in the air, I felt as if I'd been stung by a dozen wasps. Silently, I yelled my response:

Never! Not me! How dare you think I could remove the symbol of my marriage? What kind of wife do you think I am?

My friend's only mistake was that she asked too soon.

I witnessed Jack's last breath and heartbeat that summer day. I kissed his head before the funeral personnel carried him out of the house. I brought home his ashes from the mortuary and placed them in his study for the burial later. Even with all those brushes with reality, I maintained the illusion that he might walk through the front door at any moment with an explanation for his absence: *"Talle, I'm home! I forgot to tell you that I had an out-of-town conference..."* Or maybe this was a hideous nightmare and soon I would wake, shaking in his arms, hearing, *"Talle, wake up. I'm here. You're safe."* Wearing my ring sustained the delusion. *Wait for him,* the ring confirmed whenever I stared at my left hand, *you are still married.*

But thirteen months later, this wasn't a dream; it was my life, the new normal. "The Afterwards," as I called it. Every day as a widow involved dozens of questions, concerns, and decisions that rattled in my head and stirred my sleep. I frequently wondered, *What am I doing?*

and occasionally left myself breathless by taking some long-deferred action.

Thirteen months later, I stood at a jewelry store counter, shame burning up from the floor through the soles of my work shoes until my face flushed. I grasped my wedding ring and, with a slight twist and a tug over the knuckle, I pulled it off and handed it to the clerk, unable to look her in the eye.

Oh, God, what have I done?

There were three awful tasks in the thirty minutes after Jack died.

The first: the call to the hospice to tell of Jack's passing.

The second: the call to the mortuary for the removal of Jack from the house.

The third awful task was taking off Jack's wedding ring.

Hanging up the phone after the call to the mortuary, I returned upstairs to our bedroom and slipped into the bed behind his quiet body. *One last time.* I was tearless, numb, as if I, too, was floating above all of this and watching a life end.

I got out of bed from the man I loved so much. He was so still.

Come back. Don't leave me. I'm not ready to be alone.

The circulating fan in the room was the only thing that moved as I stood and stared from the foot of the bed. Maybe it was the warm breeze on my back that pushed me forward to do something, to feel useful. I grabbed the edge of the sheet and covered his exposed foot. Was I trying to keep him warm? As my left hand pulled on the sheet, the diamonds on my ring caught the light and drew my eye. My gaze snapped to his hand: *His ring!*

His ring was still on his hand, which was balled into a fist. I never thought to ask the hospice nurse how much time I had before rigor mortis set in. In my imagination, I saw a technician at the funeral home cutting off his finger to return the ring to me. I shuddered at the thought of him being mutilated. *Do something.*

I sat down next to Jack. He had rolled onto his left side after getting into bed last night, with his left arm tucked under his head, pillow-like. His hand was visible behind his head. I took his left hand, it wasn't cold, and I straightened his ring finger.

I spoke softly to him, "I'm taking your ring, Jackson. I hope that's okay."

I waited for some resistance, to hear his knuckles crackle, or for Jack to suddenly flinch, open his eyes, and complain, *Hey, what are you doin'?* But the ring slipped off easily, and I gently re-curled his ring finger to match the rest of his hand.

Holding Jack's ring was the first nudge into accepting the loss. This symbol of our marriage was heavy in my hand. I placed the ring under the light on his nightstand so I would see it every time I came into the room. *Good enough for now.*

The night before my stop at the jeweler's, in the quiet of the bathroom, I soaked my ring in a cleaning solution and worked it over with a polishing cloth. Preparation for another end, another change, as if preparing a corpse for burial. A sacred moment. The small nicks and scratches did not polish out; the ring had been worn hard over time.

Holding it in the light, the gold reflected another time from the past. I saw the day Jack held my hand, his blue-grey eyes into my brown, asking, "Will you marry me, again?" for our ninth anniversary.

He slipped the new ring onto my finger, then answered the same question as I slipped the matching ring onto his hand.

A thousand times over, yes, I will marry you again.

In the bathroom, small diamonds twinkled at me through a prism of tears. I slipped the ring back on my finger. After more than two dozen years, I had one more night with a wedding ring on my left hand.

On the way to the jeweler's the next morning, bright sun came through the windshield of Jack's Ranger truck. Although it was warm inside the cab, a shiver ran up my back and bristled the hair on my arms. I toyed with my ring, sparkles like glitter from the diagonal line of gems. These were its final moments on my left hand. An acid taste covered my tongue. My hands trembled.

Oh, Jackson, tell me I am doing the right thing. I spoke to the sky through the windshield. *Please talk to me. I needed a penny.*

I found pennies in random spots after Jack died: the middle of grocery aisles, walking trails, restaurant lobbies, even on a soccer field. Whenever I was missing him, needing confirmation of his presence, eventually a penny would show up at my feet. These coins were my last thread connecting us; he was quiet lately. No visits, no dreams, no whispers. I believed his spirit had left this realm so that I could figure out how to live on my own. But believing that didn't stop my pleas.

Help me, please. And today I had burning questions that only Jack could answer. *Are you mad at me for taking my ring off?*

There was no penny on the ground as I stepped out of the car.

I walked only five or six steps from my parking spot to the front entrance, a secured glass door with a doorbell. Someone inside spotted me and released the electronic lock. I heard the "click," pulled the door open, and stepped inside the air-conditioned foyer. Another click as the door closed behind me. Locked in like a prisoner. My lungs struggled for a breath. I wanted to bolt back to the truck, find another store, maybe in the local mall with its open doorways that invited customers to come and go without feeling like thieves. But I was in. I needed to do this while I was still willing.

The clerk's hands, covered in rings, were cupped together as she watched me from behind the counter. She sized me up the moment I pressed the bell for the security doors to open. In my paint-and-caulk-stained cutoffs and matching tank top, I wasn't dressed as if I came off the tennis courts or was headed to cocktails. She knew I wasn't buying a large emerald pendant or impressive earrings. Something simple.

"How may I help you?"

My ring suddenly felt incredibly heavy, as if its weight had rooted my feet into the red carpet. The ceiling fixtures bounced light off mirrored columns to illuminate every corner of the room.

"I would like my wedding ring resized to fit my right-hand ring finger."

I removed my ring and gave it to the clerk. Done. Vomit rose, and I swallowed hard against it. I focused on the necklaces in the case.

"There's an inscription," I muttered, swallowing the extra saliva in my mouth, "that I would like saved."

Turning the ring, she read silently and looked up with a question in her eyes.

"It's a private story. I need it saved."

The rings we wore at Jack's death weren't the first rings we exchanged. Jack's original wedding ring was a simple gold band, which eventually wore thin on the inside and needed either repair or replacement. My original set was a traditional engagement ring with a skinny wedding band attached; two years later, Jack added another band to sandwich the quarter-carat setting. The simplicity of those first rings represented a time in life, he was in his early thirties, and me in my late twenties, both teachers low on the pay scale, budgeting for child-support payments for his two sons.

The second set of matching bands was thicker and wider, and sparkled with a diagonal row of five small diamonds on Jack's and four on mine. On the inside of Jack's original and the new ring, I had inscribed, "Forever My Divine Love," along with our wedding date. I thought it would serve as a reminder of our anniversary, teasing him that the inscription gave him no excuse to forget. But the truth was, unlike some husbands, he was vigilant and thoughtful and generous throughout our almost twenty-seven years. He always remembered. We assumed we would celebrate a golden anniversary, and then onto our "Forever."

The inscription on my original ring was a joke that started early in our relationship. Four years before we met, I adopted a twelve-pound Cockapoo/Chihuahua puppy from a pet store and named her "Ms. PE Sneakers." When Jack came along, Sneaks and I teamed together and placed him under a "contract" to remain with us for infinity. Whenever Jack did something special for me, Sneakers and I conferred to determine how many more days would be added to the base of infinity.

"OK, Sneaks, that was pretty nice of Jack to bring home some carnations for me." The conference was carried out within Jack's earshot. I heard him chuckle and tried to hold a straight face and serious tone.

"I vote for another day. What do you think?" I paused, as if Sneakers was relating her opinion via those brown eyes and listening ears. "Three days? Wow, that's generous for just a dozen carnations. How about two?"

Pause.

"Yeah, I think adding two more days is good, too."

Jack protested, "Two days? That's all? Come on, Sneaks, wasn't it me that brought your last toy home?"

I snickered. "You are not a part of the negotiations, and no influence is allowed from outside parties," I scolded in my best teacher voice, disciplining Jack for his interference. Then came the laughter, hugs, kisses.

These negotiations were regular events during our twelve years as a threesome. From time to time, Jack threw out an estimate of how many days he'd stacked up, making it more complicated each time.

"I'm sure it was infinity plus seven months, two weeks, and three days."

We ceased the contract game when Sneakers was put to rest around her sixteenth birthday. The game simply didn't fit with Annie B when we adopted her a few months later. Annie B was *our* dog; Sneakers was my dog, who adopted Jack. That special tradition belonged to our beginning as a young couple, but the sentiment of the game lasted far beyond.

The inscription inside my wedding rings reads, "Infinity Plus…"

There are as many ways to deal with a wedding ring as there are widowed spouses. Wear the ring or not. Move the ring to another finger. And if not on a finger, what to do with it? There is no deadline for the decision. No rules.

Two widowed acquaintances of mine took off their wedding rings as soon as they heard the medical team declare, "She's gone," and, "He's passed."

One explained, "I am no longer married."

The other said bluntly, "Why wear a wedding ring when she's dead?"

Such a hasty decision, made amidst the chaos of death, stunned me. I had little to say in response to these stories, though I had plenty of judgment. *Do they think their marriages ended at the same hour as the lives of their loved ones? How could they think clearly at that moment?* But in another breath, I realized: let them follow their hearts, just as I needed others to respect my own difficult decisions.

My mother wore her wedding ring until her death, twenty-eight years after Dad died. Mother never considered dating or remarrying. I thought it was out of fear of loving someone again. Why put your heart and body through watching another loved one decline into death? Why go through the hell of widowhood all over again? But perhaps her commitment, *'til death do you part,* stretched beyond the grave. Dad was the only one for her, and they would be reunited in some afterlife existence. By not marrying again, Mother avoided the mess of two men meeting her at the Pearly Gates, vying for her affections. A celestial ménage à trois. What would God say about that? We might have laughed at that idea, but our relationship had been strained for years before her death, keeping us from the chuckles and empathy that could have been shared between mother and daughter. Between widows.

"I know of someone who had a jeweler melt down his ring into something else," a friend offered when I confessed that it seemed wasteful to keep Jack's ring in the safe-deposit box.

"Into what?" I sneered. What could a jeweler make that would ever capture the memories found in a wedding ring?

"Well," she ventured, "perhaps… a pendant."

"Of what?" I snapped.

"Oh, it doesn't matter. Whatever you want. It can't mean everything… It's only a piece of jewelry."

Only a piece of jewelry? My body stiffened, picturing a tacky bird or a clumsy clump of gold made from Jack's wedding ring, hanging from a chain around my neck. Ludicrous. Sacrilegious. Melting that ring would be like ripping out chapters of a rare book, folding them into paper airplanes, and saying, "It's only a bunch of pages."

I considered putting Jack's wedding ring on a sturdy golden chain, long enough so the ring would tap its presence on my chest, like someone rapping on the window to be let in. But I knew a cold metallic thump would not offer any solace or peace when I craved his voice. For the moment, I kept Jack's ring intact and safe inside the bank. It would stay there until I found an option I could live with.

The ringless finger made me feel lopsided, like being shoeless on one foot, walking with an irregular gait. I had all kinds of irrational thoughts: Better to lose the left ring finger or the entire left hand. An amputation accident would lay the responsibility elsewhere, on fate or God, but not on me. By removing that ring from my left hand, I had transformed myself from Jack's wife to a widow and a single woman. I felt treasonous.

I still had that reservation for the ten-day Eastern Mediterranean cruise. The details were in a well-marked file folder on a corner of my desk. The cruise represented, now that I was alone, a new future, away from this house and the life I'd lived in it. This would be my first time in Europe, an adventure once planned together. This was my chance to overcome the fear of being a single woman traveling alone. I would travel from Seattle to Barcelona, sleeping on a twin bed in a small hotel. I would walk to the departure dock, dragging my new luggage, setting off to visit seven coastal cities in five countries. I would spend time alone in new lands, without the language skills or knowledge of money or food, or customs. Imagining all of it, I felt guilty for doing this without Jack. I felt excited, fearful, and intimidated. I wanted to prove to myself that I could do this.

My widow's mantras knocked inside my skull.

If not now, when?

Get the first time out of the way; the second time will be easier. If not the second time, then the one after that. Keep going until it is easier.

But I needed to take off my wedding ring. I wanted to be free to date on the ship, to be unobserved by anyone who knew me, knew Jack, knew us. I needed anonymity to protect myself from the shame I felt for wanting to touch another man. I wanted no judgments from those who knew my story. If I wore my wedding ring, any man who didn't respect it wasn't a man for me, even if it was just a ten-day cruise-ship romance. I could only embark on a new phase of my life if the ring was off. Logic, pure and simple.

I had taken pages out of our wedding book, folded them into paper airplanes, and tossed them into the wind.

Chapter 16
Questions: A Cruise Alone and Dating a Passenger

A cruise ship romance, a passionate kiss, only fifteen months after Jack's death. What was I thinking?

After a late evening show and stroll on the upper deck of the ship, did this new man, this not-complete stranger, feel my confusion during our first embrace? How did my lips send no message to go further? How I held his shoulders as if they were the ship railing? His hands on my back, his warm breath on my face, his touches failed to arouse a deep yearning. Not even a stir. As our tongues met, my mind sprang to action, reminding myself:

I'm not cheating. I'm not cheating.

My vows are null and void.

Jack's dead. I'm widowed.

In the last twenty-eight years, I hadn't French-kissed anyone but Jack. Our tongues knew how to dance with each other, how to set off a deeper desire. But that chorus of reminders, I'm not cheating, did not drown out the loud, slow drumbeat response that came.

I am still Jack's wife.

I was the first of my five siblings, soccer teammates, former colleagues, and close friends to be widowed. I had no one to guide me through "The Afterwards." Although many loved Jack and grieved his death with me, they could only imagine losing their own partner. I knew to my marrow the agony of loss, and I knew it alone.

Two months before the cruise trip, my brother Mark left a voice message: "I want to be the first one today to say I love you."

Although his words were intended as a warmhearted gesture, I shook my head and bellowed at the machine. "Because you, Mark, *are the only one*, the only one who will say that to me today! Or tomorrow." From a fearful corner of my heart, "Or ever."

Maybe this solo life was what I would have until my own death. Could I live with that? Fifteen months was too soon to know, but the shadow loomed.

Right up to the day I handed over the keys to the new owner of our house, I'd heard Jack's "I don't love you; I *adore* you," from the walls. I felt his gentle caresses on the small of my back, nibbles on the neck, and massages of tight shoulders. That glow, that tingling, the lightness of heart, and the stir of energy that came from being adored. "I adore you" was the standard for any man in my future. I wouldn't settle for less.

It was hard to fathom, could I let my body feel sexually alive again? Would another man's hand feel abrasive in mine? Would another's kiss curdle in my mouth? Would I be punished with guilt if another man's eyes held my gaze, let myself be enveloped in his arms, and let him fill the emptiness I held? Would I later regret not trudging through the muck of the pain and loneliness a little longer and not rush into something new?

Between the loss of appetite, preparing the house for the real estate market, and all the hustling the quick sale required, my body was leaner. Shopping for clothes to wear for the trip, the unfamiliar woman staring back from the dressing room mirrors wasn't the person who married Jack. I owned the smile wrinkles and the crow's feet, the eyebrow skin that drooped more towards the eyelids. My upper arms, particularly the backsides, stubbornly resisted the toning exercises; I was slowly acquiring my "squirrel wings." But with a good hairstylist and monthly re-coloring, I still appeared younger than my mid-fifties. The inner clock agreed.

I was an immigrant to the world of dating and always had been. Even as an adolescent. I was a lousy dancer, never learned or played the dating games, struggled to understand their rules, and abhorred the premise that my feminine role was "focusing on the interests of the male." (Thank you, Mother, for that inane advice.) I neither flirted well nor felt comfortable using people for free meals. Besides, I loved simple tavern fare and *one* drink. As I often teased Jack, "I'm cheap, but not easy."

My plan for the ship romance was premeditated and callous. I'd seek out an eligible man who was close to my age, pleasant to look at, and showed interest in me. I would enjoy his company, then leave all of it, the romance and man, behind at the last port. I knew I would be using him. It was not my style to lead someone on, and I struggled to accept this new part of me that would do so. I didn't see how else to go about it, as I was not looking for a commitment or long-term relationship. Just dipping a toe into the deep end of the pool for a possible future swim.

This ship was a safe and secluded place with no family or friends on board. A small town-at-sea, a new neighborhood where no one knew me, where I packed away the widow's black and reinvented myself for ten days. Here, I needn't defend a new man sitting next to me, nor see the judgmental looks of *Isn't it a bit too soon?* I was already asking that question myself.

My mother had promised not to be with anyone after her husband's death. Didn't I love Jack as deeply as she did Dad? Why shouldn't I make that promise, too? I knew I wasn't my mother, of course, I would make different choices than she did, but the truth was, even thinking about another man felt like a betrayal. An affair. I still felt married inside and out; committed to Jack, like a second skin I could not shed. I'd worn it so long, so faithfully, and it fitted so well. Or once did. But lately, it hung unevenly at an edge or two, a ripped hem of a beloved overcoat, threadbare at the elbows and cuffs, still providing warmth, but showing age. The plan felt so strange, but *if not now, when?* The passengers of this ship would not have condemning eyes, would not care to witness my awkwardness. This was my chance.

A claustrophobe would never pick this room for a ten-day cruise. Located on the lowest deck, in the bowels of the ship, the room was small and windowless, the cheapest option available. Regardless of the time of day, I left the small wall sconces on. The queen bed, wedged between two built-in nightstands, filled half the room. In the other half was a corner closet and the bathroom, which could not be entered if the closet doors were opened. After being outside in the fresh breeze of the upper deck, this room held stale air. Having sold my house just days before the cruise, and when I returned to the States, I would begin the hunt for a new residence. For now, this tiny room was my home.

Each time a room steward visited for evening turn-down service, the golden satin bedspread was pulled to the foot of the bed, the pale-yellow blanket and ironed white sheet were folded back into a wrinkle-less triangle on the left and right sides, a bath towel folded into an origami animal sat in the middle, and chocolate mints on the pillows punctuated the whole picture.

I still used only the left side of the bed regardless of where I slept: home, a friend's guest room, the cabin, or a hotel. The right was Jack's side, still. Three days into the trip, the room steward noticed: he turned down the left half of the bed, leaving the right intact, with only one mint.

I returned to my room for sleep, dressing, and refuge, especially when the sight of couples holding hands, talking, and laughing over meals shattered my resolve to get through this, to have fun. At these moments, I missed Jack too deeply and needed to fold into a ball on the floor and weep.

Hey, someone! Talk to me. I have a good sense of humor. I'm a good listener.

I found that, in most cases, I had to start the small talk. Most people were traveling in pairs or in groups, which excluded new members. No one just walked up to me with a simple "*Hi*." The most I got from strangers were words of necessity and manners: "Excuse me" in the buffet line, "Which floor?" in the elevator, or "Can we get by, please?" when I stopped to read information posted on the walls.

At my first morning breakfast, I was determined to wade into conversation. I'd adjusted to a quiet life back in Washington but was immediately overwhelmed by noise in the large dining area. There were so many people, so many languages, so much clattering of plates and cups. So many comings and goings. I felt I was in the chaos of the Seattle Folk Life Festival or IKEA's yearly sale, with little room to walk or find a comfortable spot for sitting. People were yelling across the way to each other: "Over here!" as they grabbed a clean vacant table, or "Get me some of that, too," to a friend standing in line. And there was so much food, everywhere. An omelet bar sizzled with fried onions and diced ham or bacon pieces. Varieties of pastries and breads of all sizes lined up neatly on tray after tray next to colorful fresh strawberries, pineapple, grapes, and kiwi. Children's eyes were wide at the options; their plates were as overfilled as their parents'.

I wished for a "Singles Sit Here" section, a safe place to start new friendships without inspecting for wedding bands first. This first meal would set the tone for the trip. I wanted to meet new people, perhaps he's in this room? With a tray in hand, I found an older couple eating at a table meant for four; there were few open spaces. *Safe start,* I thought. Pointing to the empty chair at their table, I asked, "May I join you?" Nodding, they continued to chew their meals.

"Have you been on a cruise before?" My question resulted in blank stares, the rapid fire of words in another language between them, and a rocky, "No English." What were the chances, when there were three thousand people aboard this ship, that I chose a couple who did not speak English? Do I stay and quickly consume my oatmeal and hard-boiled egg, making my presence awkward for them, or slither away to an empty table, making my absence awkward for them? I smiled, nodded my head, and ate quickly in their silence. The following days, I ate breakfast by a corner window, "Me and the Sea" for the rest of the trip. I had only one dart of courage in my arsenal, and I had missed the board.

On the second night at sea, sailing from Barcelona, Spain, to Nicé, France, dinner was a dress-up night: men in tuxes or fine three-piece suits, and women in gowns or elegant cocktail dresses. My hair was done, makeup on, and three diamonds, graded in size, decorated each earlobe. The smallest stud on my left ear was the diamond I had removed from my original engagement ring just a few months prior to this trip. It matched the stud in the right lobe that I bought when I passed my exams for my master's degree twenty years ago. Two more sets finished the line of glitter. If nothing else, my ears sparkled rich and sophisticated.

I opened my cabin door into the narrow hallway and felt immediately pressed back into the room by a rush of sound, people leaving for dinner, voices of all ages.

"Follow me, I know where we're seated."

"Do you have the room key?"

"Roger, no running in the halls."

I had never been comfortable in social situations where I knew no one, but I did have my Irish wit to ease the way; I couldn't stifle a humorous retort or comment if I tried. All I needed was a willing audience to laugh with me. Working with adolescents, parents, and school staff for so many years, conversation starters were easy. Keeping the conversation going, especially with strangers, was the challenge.

I took a deep breath and released a long exhale.

"Come on, Meryl, here we go," I told myself, stepping out of my cabin into the river of passengers. I'd decided to tap into the persona of Meryl Streep in "*The Devil Wears Prada*". Who would mess with Miranda Priestly? Crowds would part, doors would open, a chair would be pulled out, and a fine Malbec poured as Meryl sat down. *Yeah, Meryl and I.*

Holding my head high, shoulders back, an embroidered shawl over my forearm, anticipating a chilly walk in the sea air that evening, I strolled past the cocktail lounges with live music trios, where glasses clinked, laughter erupted, and couples moved on the small dance floors. I steered myself toward the soft classical music and formality of the dining room in the stern.

I felt eyes following me and felt flattered, but uncertain what to do next. I could never walk up to a staring man and ask him to dance. Besides, who was I kidding? I wanted to feel gorgeous and sexy, but in truth, those men were checking out a lonely older woman in a sharply tailored black cocktail dress.

I was ill-prepared for the elegance of the dining room, especially after months of eating quick and easy meals back home, popping popcorn for dinner because I didn't have the energy for anything more elaborate, and rarely changing out of my shorts and T-shirt. Tonight, I sat at a circular table with pressed white linens, fine glassware, and a variety of forks, spoons, and knives. The table was set for three couples, two of whom were already seated and chatting. My tablemates were twenty or so years older than I, with their silvered hair, liver-spotted hands, and warm, welcoming smiles. After we exchanged names and home cities (Margaret and Bill of London, Irene and Peter of Edinburgh, Tally from Seattle), the empty chair beside me begged to be introduced.

"Traveling alone?" Margaret asked.

All eyes turned to me. Under the table, I twirled my wedding ring, exiled to my right hand, and pictured Jack's matching ring, still stored in the safe-deposit box. On my left hand, middle finger, was a new ring I'd purchased on my annual beach trip this year. How glad I was to be distracted from the unfamiliar nakedness of my left ring finger.

Oh, damn it, Jack, you should be in that chair.

I hadn't anticipated the empty chair, nor rehearsed any lines to explain my solo status. Words tumbled in my head. I didn't want pity. I didn't want to explain four years of cancer treatments, remissions, and his death. I wanted to say the truth, but without crying. They waited.

"Yes, I am." I paused and took a breath. "My husband passed from cancer fifteen months ago. This cruise was supposed to be a celebration of our twenty-seventh wedding anniversary last year. I'm fulfilling our dream."

I didn't tell them about the travel brochures that Jack and I collected, my handwritten notes from two presentations on Greek travel, or my plan to toast to our twenty-eighth wedding anniversary en route to Athens. Yes, I was traveling alone, but, of course, I brought Jack with me.

My reply stopped the conversation, most people don't know how to respond. Before them sat a relatively young widow, younger than they. I was what they feared becoming: alone, left behind, living uncoupled. I used my pro chitchat skills to divert the conversation from myself, and the evening carried on. By the third night of the cruise, the extra place setting and chair were gone when I arrived for dinner.

On a tour four days later, in the parked bus, I waited for the slower walkers to return from a half-mile hike to the top of a crater. An easy walk. Two men sat down in the row ahead of me seconds after I sat. Turning my attention to the trailhead out the window, I reflected on the beauty and history I had seen.

What do you think of that big hole, Jackson? Pretty cool, huh?

I thought of Jack's knees, both needing eventual replacement, and whether he could have made the climb. I wondered if he'd be one of the last ones on the bus.

If you were with me, Bubba, would we have picked a different excursion or toughed it out?

The sun blasted through the windows on our side of the bus. Over the top of the tall navy seatback ahead of me floated, "Do you mind if we close these drapes?"

With his accent, this stranger's words made a serenade of a simple question. He could have recited nursery rhymes, and I would have enthusiastically stood and asked for an encore.

"Sure, no problem." I pulled the cloth drape from my window toward him, and he grabbed the edge to shade his seat. Raising the clear plastic water bottle I bought before going ashore, tilting it toward his very red, very sweaty face, I asked, "Could you use some water?"

His companion on the aisle side of the row jumped in with the same singing accent. "I brought some for both of us," he said, flashing a bottle over the top of the seat at me. I saw a sliver of his face through the space between the seats. White hair. Smiling.

It was time to make good use of my forte, easy, noncommittal conversation, the way I would talk to strangers in the checkout line at the local grocery store about the weather, local sports teams, or the cost of out-of-season fruit.

"Where are you boys from?"

"Scotland. And you?"

"The States." I had learned from European passengers that the answer wasn't "The United States," "The U.S.," or "America."

I saw his head shift left then right, eyeing the empty seat next to me. "Traveling alone?"

That damn question. I wanted to snip, *No shit, Sherlock,* but I knew empty seats provoked curiosity. Tablemate Margaret taught me that.

"Yes." I saw his eyebrows arch, so I turned toward the window and feigned interest in the stragglers getting on the bus. Behind my sunglasses, my vision clouded. My lips pinched together to hold in the cry of grief rising from my chest.

"No one's traveling with you?" he nudged again.

I drew a deep breath. Of course, he didn't know. Maybe his questions were meant to be small talk, breezy.

I unclenched my jaw, sniffled, and said, "My husband and I were going to do this cruise last year before he..." I let the sentence float off and turned my head back to the window, biting my lower lip.

The stranger quickly filled the space left by my unfinished sentence. "I lost my wife four years ago. Neil's wife died just three months ago." All three of us were widowed, magnets pulled together by the synergy of grief.

Is this God telling me I'm not alone?

We exchanged condolences, then names. "I'm Will, this is Neil."

"I'm Tally. Good to meet you." That was all. We kept to our own thoughts on the route back to the ship.

In the midday sun, I lounged by the ship's wading pool, tanning in a black bikini with a lemonade-iced-tea mix sweating in its glass, a daily crossword puzzle on my lap. At one of the several outdoor food kitchens, a cook prepared American-style hamburgers for hungry tourists returning from onshore activities. The aroma of charred beef and greasy fries carried on the sea breeze across the deck but did nothing for my appetite. I chuckled to think that Jack, a healthy Jack, would have been in line, grinning like an adolescent kid as he mounded condiments upon condiments, a pile so high that he couldn't chomp both top and bottom bun in one bite, a gooey mess dripping out of his hands onto the plate. He would have eaten it all, washed his hands, and gone back for seconds in a couple of hours.

I felt a light tap on my toes and was surprised to see the Boys of Scotland standing in front of me with a bucket of chilled beers, dressed in fresh shorts and polo shirts. Neil had a full head of brunette hair cut short above his black-rimmed sunglasses; he was taller than Will by a head and thinner by fifteen pounds or so. Will tilted his sunglasses down as he passed my chair, giving me a smiling once-over. I felt naked, wanting to reach for my cover-up, yet I had brought the suit to wear it. *Stay with me here, Meryl.*

The boys plopped onto the two vacant lounge chairs on my right, Will in the closest one. Neil seemed to follow Will around like a lost little brother, still in the survival mode of early widowhood, probably surprised that he had gotten out of bed to leave the comforts of his home. Now, Neil seemed like a third wheel and leaned back in his chair to let Will engage me in conversation.

Oh, my, it's really happening; someone is interested in me.

He wasn't Jack, this Will. A nice guy, but no sparks between us like Jack and I had on our first date. Would this guy do? Could I do this?

"Smile. You can do this, Meryl," I whispered in my head.

"How did you like the crater?" Will inquired. He pushed his sunglasses up into a full head of white hair, neatly combed and parted, and peered down at me. He had a bulbous nose with a strong square jawline and ruddy complexion, my physical stereotype of a Scotsman. He could have passed as a clean-shaven, slimmer version of Santa

Claus. Neil drew a beer out of the metal bucket and passed it to Will, who, in turn, offered it to me. His knobby knuckles, the beginning of arthritis, were evidence of a man who had done some hard labor. I shook my head, picked up my plastic cup of iced tea, and tipped it toward him. Both men took long gulps of their beers.

"I like geology, so it was interesting. And you two?"

Keep both engaged; don't focus on one.

I was on an unfamiliar path, entering the dating market again after almost twenty-seven years. A woman in her fifties. Gads, I ain't any different now than when I was a teen.

"I liked it," Will said.

"How about you, Neil?" I leaned forward in my chair to look past Will.

Neil appeared hypnotized by the shimmering of the water and the voices rising from the pool. I knew what those eyes saw: another pool, a healthy wife. He heard the shared laughter, felt the wet of her skin, like silk, on his. His film of memories was running, projected over the day.

"Oh, pardon me, what did you say?" he asked, startled.

"How did you like the crater trip?" Will repeated.

"Fine, just fine," he said, and his eyes returned to the pool.

I drew him back, taking a risk. "Neil, what caused her death?"

I tossed aside my tourist cap and used my chops as a school counselor: engage him, let him process by telling the story, and help him for a few minutes without pushing too hard.

Speaking to his hands, Neil said, "Cancer. Breast cancer."

"Excuse my French, gentlemen," I said, looking back and forth between them. "Fuck cancer."

Will's eyebrows rose, and Neil's shoulders stiffened. The Boys of Scotland raised their eyebrows. Any refinement they saw in me had been tossed overboard with that comment, I guessed.

"I lost Jack to cancer, too. Skin cancer. So, I earned that profanity."

Will smiled. "Yeah, cancer's a bugger, all right. Like Neil, I lost my wife to breast cancer."

"You're pretty amazing, Neil, to leave the house so soon. I could never do this trip after three months."

Will jumped in. "Neil has been a friend for a long time. I dragged him out to get some fresh air," and he patted Neil's knee. Neil tipped his head toward his friend, then returned his gaze to the pool.

Three months. What was I doing three months after Jack's death? My mind was blank. End of September: no school, entering my second year of retirement. I survived, obviously. The dog was fed and walked, the house didn't burn down, and I didn't cause a car accident. I held it together, but how? I could only remember the overwhelming mounds of paperwork, dropping Jack's ashes off a ferry into Puget Sound, and the Celebration of Life with over three hundred people. And the daily crying bouts. Nothing more. All those months of day-to-day living were erased.

It had grown quiet between the three of us. *Think of something to say, Tally, and not about the weather.*

"What are you doing tomorrow?" I turned to both.

Will answered, they had no interest in Mikonos and were staying on the ship to rest up. I wanted to walk the town alone, not part of any set excursion, determined to have a real Greek gyro with real Greek tzatziki sauce. I didn't want company.

"Well, boys, I'm off." I grabbed my wrap and, while still sitting, slipped it over my head to avoid giving an eye-level full-butt-in-bikini view to these sitters. "See you around."

"What dinner shift do you have?" Will blurted out as I stood. The ship had three dinner times.

"First." I stood over them, slipped on my pool flip-flops, and reached down for my drink.

"We do, too," Will said, flicking at Neil, then back at me. "Where are you seated?"

"Up front, just inside the door. And you?"

Look cool, calm. Breathe. Oh, Meryl.

"Way in the back."

Please don't stop by my table and say hi, I thought. I didn't want to explain this man to my tablemates when only four nights ago I was explaining widowhood. I don't want to look like a single woman desperate for a man.

"Do you go to the show afterwards?" Will asked. He was trying to link up.

Oh, this is really happening.

"Why, yes, I do. I've enjoyed them thus far." My heart raced. My mouth went dry.

Ask him something, Talle. He's doing all the work here. I took a sip of my drink, stalling, but before I could form a thought, Will continued.

"We sit on the left side in the middle balcony. Come join us." His voice carried the insecurities of a high school sophomore asking a senior to the prom.

"Okay, I'll meet you there. See ya, boys."

The rest of the day, I felt frantic. Someone was interested in me. I hadn't schemed any steps beyond this moment. I didn't think it would even happen, or at least not this easily. I hadn't thought any man would find me attractive as Jack did. But why not? My little sister was always considered the beauty of the family, with numerous boyfriends. Why not me?

After dinner, I walked to the theatre, my heart pounding in my ears.

Are you ready for this, Talle? You can do this. It might be fun.

I sat in the middle of the upper-level balcony and looked down, scanning for a white-haired man sitting with a brunette male companion on the left side. I didn't see them. The longer I tried, the more I lost my nerve. I gave up when the house lights were turned down and slipped out immediately after the show was over, heading back to my room.

Chicken.

The next day, in Croatia, I bumped into Will, Neil, and two new friends of theirs at an in-port excursion. My tour of a historical castle in Split was beginning as theirs was ending.

"We missed you at the show." Will's smile sent a twinkle into his eyes, and his face flushed.

"I was there and didn't see you. I guess I wasn't clear exactly where you would be seated."

"I have an idea."

Oh, I bet you do.

"Meet us at the upper port side door after dinner. We'll get you seated properly."

After dinner, I walked the length of the ship, and panic rose with each step. What the hell was I doing? Will could be a creep in nice clothes. A stalker whom I'd have to avoid for the rest of the trip, ducking in and out of crowds.

Meryl, hope you're packing some pepper spray, because I left mine at home.

I waited at the theater entrance for several minutes. Had Will chickened out like I did the night before? With each passing minute, my heart raced faster and faster.

Are you really ready for this?

I paced back and forth in a small nearby art gallery with a clear view of the hallway and was just about to give up and return to my upper-tier seat when I saw them.

OK, Meryl, here we go.

Will wasn't Jack, and I craved the familiarity of that twenty-seven-year friendship. I wanted Jack next to me to talk about all the things we had in common besides a day on a cruise ship. I wanted years of warm memories. I didn't want to work to sustain a conversation. I wanted shared silences to be smooth and accepting, not awkward bumps in the road. As we waited for the start of the show, our chitchat was stiff, and topics of conversation often sank into short answers.

"Do you have any pets?" I asked.

"No, too much work," he said.

Silence.

"I love dogs. I had to put a fifteen-year-old, fifty-pound Shepherd mix to rest four months ago, and I plan on another furry friend in my life when I return." His eyes wandered off to the crowd.

More silence.

"Do you have a home or an apartment?" I asked.

"A house. Small one with a small yard. Just enough for a few flowers and easy care. I've been there for thirty-five years."

"I sold my house a few days ago." "*My house*" soured in my mouth. I thought of it still as *ours*. "So, when I return to the States, I'll sleep in friends' spare rooms for doctor appointments and socialization with friends, staying mostly at the cabin two hours away until I find a new house to buy."

"Don't rush into anything. Give yourself time," he advised. "Maybe a condo?" *He's not listening to my needs. Does he have his own agenda?*

"Nah, I need dirt under my nails from a garden. What flowers do you like?"

A light conversation, poking into commonalities and differences. Will had never moved from the house he shared with his late wife; I sold mine. He had a son; I had two stepsons, whose relationships with me were quite cool. Will was a salesman with a high school diploma, and I was a school counselor with two college degrees. Neither one of us was sure how to tease without being too forward or too personal.

His arm around my shoulders at the show sent shivers down my back. Jack would have simply held my hand, knowing I favored that touch. I was unsure about Will's arm and kept my hands on my lap.

What message am I sending by doing nothing?

Afterward, we walked down the stairs and down the hallway to my cabin door. After I retrieved my door card from my purse, I turned to face him.

"Good night," I said.

Will stepped toward me and placed a light kiss on my cheek. "Tomorrow?"

"See you then." I turned and quickly entered my room. He wanted to see me again. I couldn't help but wonder why.

On my bedstand was a framed picture of Jack. I grabbed it, rocked on the edge of the bed with the metal frame pressed into my chest.

I miss you, I miss you, I miss you. With a deep sigh, I pulled the photo back and looked into Jack's eyes.

Are you OK with this, Jackson? I'm widowed, and you are gone, but it feels like I am cheating on you. Like I should grieve the rest of my life for how much I love you. No one could ever match you and what you gave to me. What am I doing?

Amidst the muffled hum of the ship engines, Jack smiled from the photo. A single mint sat on the pillow on the left side of the bed.

At the show the next night, Will's arm wrapped around me again, and his fingers softly massaged my shoulder. Perhaps his wife liked this, but I wasn't thrilled. Afterward, on the promenade, Will bought two plastic cups of good red wine from an outdoor bar. We walked under a full moon, lots of stars, and I wished I felt aroused instead of weary.

Will was a kind man, but our conversation felt mentally draining, awkward. As we talked about the different excursions we took that day, the show, and what each of us ordered for dinner, I had fallen in love with escargot. I double-checked and rethought what I said, speaking with a restraint that was rarely necessary between Jack and me. Will's laughter wasn't as giggly as Jack's, more reserved, like how one laughed politely after hearing a joke for the second time. Maybe I wasn't as witty as Jack made me feel.

One would think suffering through our spouses' deaths would give us much to share and compare. But no. Will held his grief and memories tight to himself, like an over-cinched belt.

"How are you doing now, after four years without your wife?"

"Just fine." His short answer and not asking me about my grief ended the conversation. Thereafter, we did not talk about our losses in any detail and kept the tone light and safe.

Repeatedly, I had to remind myself: There was only one Jack Reynolds.

Surprisingly, I was Will's first dating experience after his wife's death. It's a man's world in the senior dating scene, single women outnumber men, and Will was handsome enough, courteous, and an attentive listener. Well-trained by his late wife, I chuckled to myself.

"So, I've got to know. Why aren't you dating, Will?" I asked, taking a sip of wine. "Surely, Scottish women have knocked on the door with casseroles and cakes."

He leaned over the rail, eyeing the waves below. "I wasn't ready."

"Really? There's been no one?"

Turning toward me, he said, "A few friends at the church stopped by, but..." and dropped his eyes to his well-polished shoes. "No, nothing serious. Just wasn't ready."

The wall around this topic rose between us, and I never pressed for more. "*I wasn't ready*" was my own answer to so many questions. I, too, leaned over the railing and watched the prow cut white-crested waves out into the otherwise calm sea.

"My doctor gave me a clean bill of health last month. He said that I'm as fit as a forty-five-year-old." He peeked sideways at me. "Good heart, good lungs."

Into his gray-blue eyes, under those snow-colored eyebrows, I wanted to ask, "*Why are you telling me about your doctor visit?*

Oh, do the math, Tally. You're fifty-six and he's sixty-eight. Twelve years difference.

Would that gap be too much for me? Is he looking for a nurse for his old age, knowing the statistical likelihood that I would outlive him? I didn't want to reenter the hell of widowhood any time soon. Months earlier, at an event sponsored by my widowed support group, an eighty-something-year-old widower friend gave sound advice:

"You're a real catch, Tally. Be careful. Ya got a pension, and some men only want a nurse-with-a-purse." Back then, I smiled, confused, and thanked him. But tonight, with Will's age and health proclamations, I understood a little better.

"That's great, Will," I said, and he went on to talk about his exercise routine of daily walks and weightlifting. *Was he trying to sell himself as a good match?*

My plan was a simple ship romance, an experiment, nothing about "forever." My gut twisted as I considered for the first time that Will might have something else in mind. Was I playing a game with a man's heart? Was he going to be hurt? Who knew he would be so eager to be coupled again, with a woman he hardly knew? Or did he come on board with a plan, too?

I began backstepping. "Did I mention that I played soccer? I jog regularly so I can play. I'm missing a game this week. I'm sure my team is anxious for my return." How choppy my sentences sounded. I had to make sure he understood that I was headed back to the States, *without him.* "Scotland is a tad behind the States with its women's sports, isn't it?"

Will sputtered, "It's not that bad. Really. They're working on it. They'll get better."

Had I hit a nerve? I went another direction. "Tell me about your house, your yard. What's the neighborhood like? I only ask because real estate is on my mind. I'm eager to return home and purchase my own new home."

Could I be any clearer?

Will spoke about a cottage-like home, a few bedrooms, and a small, low-maintenance yard. Then he added, "Don't rush into buying anything. A house can be a lot of work. Give yourself some time to travel. Perhaps visit Scotland?"

We both knew a mortgage payment would anchor me in the States. *He wants me in Scotland. He's discouraging my dreams. Gads, he's going way too fast. Will I be like him, desperate for a partner, when I am four years out from Jack's death and still alone?*

"I want a house with enough yard for gardens and a dog," I went on without commenting on a Scotland visit. I talked about the vegetable garden at the cabin: the abundance of tomatoes, zucchinis, pumpkins, and radishes.

"A dog? That will tie you down," he said, shaking his head.

He didn't get me or my passions. "I will always have a dog in my life," I said firmly. That was never going to change. His eyes widened, but he remained quiet.

He wasn't Jack. Jack would never ask me to live without a "four-pedder" in the house.

We walked back to my cabin in silence.

I wasn't ready for Will's passionate kiss outside my cabin door, although I knew we would get there eventually. I played along, curious about what it would be like to kiss this man. Any man. There was no standing on tiptoes to reach his lips, like I had to with Jack. I lingered in Will's arms, my hands on his broad shoulders. I inhaled the starch of his crisp white shirt under the tailored charcoal suit coat that hid his middle-aged spread. His smart blood-red tie and matching handkerchief, silk, no doubt, finished his attire in style, along with those well-polished brogues. I detected no tobacco residue, *thank God*, just a clean, musky smell.

He wasn't Jack, who would have worn his signature lime cologne.

I was not aroused, not truly enjoying the kiss. Will was an aggressive kisser, not soft or playful. He didn't kiss like Jack.

"What's wrong with American men that you aren't seeing anyone?" Will asked one afternoon on the pool deck after our separate in-port adventures. I was back in my black bikini with an iced tea, Will in a fresh cream-colored polo, navy shorts, sturdy leather sandals on his feet, and a beer in hand.

"I haven't made myself available and, like you, I am not ready." I knew that now.

I know that because of you, Will.

Will nodded his head. He knew "not ready."

I understood then, too, how cruise romances got serious quickly. I saw one person three to four times a day, for an hour to several hours at a time. Multiply that by four days, and we had gone on sixteen dates. What would have been different if we were in the same town together?

We had four days of dinner shows, walks on the promenade deck at night, and daytime conversations on the pool deck that went down like skim milk, with little flavor or depth. No sex, I wasn't ready, at least not with Will. He wasn't the right man for anything but a casual friendship, and I knew it.

On the final night on board, I got a serious migraine that demanded I skip the show to lie in the darkness of my cabin. I set an alarm and got up at what I guessed would be the curtain call, and caught Will at the exit door.

"Sorry, got a migraine and needed quiet," I explained. We walked to a nearby red velvet couch and sat.

His brow creased. "Can I get you anything? You look so sick." My face was ashen from the pain. This was an obvious ailment, and not some ploy of avoidance.

"No, sadly. The only way to break it is with darkness, quiet, and a long rest."

I wanted to have a *good* final conversation that would tie this relationship up neatly, and God knows I wanted clarity. But before I could find the words or strength, Will jumped in.

"Don't buy the dog or the house," he said, holding both my hands in his, eyes peering deeply into mine. "Please."

My heart wasn't in a future with him. He was a friend, that was all. A man who breached my solitude and showed me that I wasn't too damaged to make a connection. I hoped I'd done the same for him.

"I'm sorry. I'm going home to the States, Will. I'll see you in the morning. We'll talk more then." I placed a small kiss on his cheek and turned down the hallway to the darkness of my room. My headache demanded a quick exit.

The migraine broke sometime in the night. The next morning, I walked the deck to the gangplank and off the ship at the port of exit: Venice. I searched around for a white-haired head bobbing in the crowd, wanting a better goodbye. When I didn't see Will, I hopped on one of the buses headed for the Venice airport. I peered out the window, hoping to catch a final glimpse of him, but I only saw strangers.

The airport smelled like the streets and canals of Venice, old and tired. Just inside the door, I spotted Will and Neil seated at a small café at a table for two. I walked over and smiled at them both.

"I thought I'd missed the chance for a final goodbye. I've been on the lookout for you two all morning," I said.

Will's face showed his exhaustion: drawn, pale, drained of his usual enthusiasm. But he managed a grin. Neil got up and motioned for me to sit in his chair. "Can I get you something to drink?"

"I would love a tea, Neil. Thank you," I said.

"Make it two," Will added.

Neil left for the tea, and I turned to Will. "This is it, Will. I'm heading home and you to yours."

His head nodded. Silence.

"I want to thank you for everything."

You're sounding pretty corny, Talle.

"You look really tired. Are you okay?"

The rings under his eyes said it all. "I am a bit. Rough night of sleep."

Neil returned holding three paper cups of brown, tepid water, placed two cups on the table, and left with his. The overhead speaker announced boarding gates every few minutes; we both lent it half an ear. The Boys of Scotland were off to Edinburgh, a relatively short flight. I had the long hops from Venice to London to New York to Chicago to Seattle.

The café table reminded me of the schoolrooms of my youth, chrome legs, wobbly and uneven beneath us as we shifted through a difficult conversation. I covered Will's hands on the table with mine, trying to look into his downcast eyes.

"You're asking me to give up my country and my friends, Will. I wouldn't ask that of you, insisting you come to the States to live. You love Scotland, and I love the U.S."

"But you can go back and visit as much as you like," he said, looking up. He offered a compromise and tried to poke cracks in my thinking.

"You know that wouldn't be enough for either one of us."

And you are not what I want.

Tears filled his eyes. He knew.

I gathered my words. "Thank you for making me feel beautiful again. I will always have a special place in my heart for you, Will. Always. If I must, I'll come to Scotland and yell at you for not dating. You're a good man. She's out there. Let her in. Like you did with me."

He nodded. His eyes shifted: no longer focused on mine, but down at our hands.

"Flight number 3476 to London boarding at gate 5," came from the overhead speakers.

"That's me." I stood up, slid my hands off his. I went around the small table, wrapped an arm around his shoulders, and gave him a squeeze and a light kiss on his cheek. "I'll be in Scotland someday," I whispered into his ear. "You'd better have a woman friend by then. You hear me?"

"I'll try." His voice sounded flat, far off.

Standing behind him, I was glad that I couldn't see his eyes. The sound of his sorrow and the slump of his shoulders were enough for me.

I am so sorry I hurt you. Where are those words, Talle?

I didn't want him to think he was a pawn in a game, that I could be that cruel. I walked away feeling ashamed of what I did, who I was.

I sought out Neil, who was pretending interest at a postcard kiosk outside the gift shop. I held up my arms, and he bent over to loop his lightly around me. Standing on tiptoe, I was the one who hugged him tighter, telling him, "You take care of yourself. It's a long road ahead."

Neil bowed his head and said a faint, "Goodbye."

I looked back at the table where Will still sat and waved to the man who thought I was beautiful. He raised his hand from the table and gave a small gesture of farewell.

"Are you excited to go home?" the woman in the adjacent seat asked me on the plane.

What home? I thought.

I laughed inside. I didn't have a house to go to; the new owner lived in the only home I really knew. My possessions were either in storage or at the cabin. I'd camp out at the cabin through winter until I found a new place in the Seattle area in the spring. I would begin opening animal rescue sites to see which dog would jump from the screen into my heart. The person picking me up at the airport on the other side of this journey would be the husband of a dear friend. Not Jack. I'd spend the night with my friends, then head to the cabin.

"Yes, I am. I am excited to go back home."

Chapter 17
Later: A New Home and Neighborhood

On a rare dry January afternoon in the Pacific Northwest, I met Lisa from across the street, and I didn't even know her last name, at our street-side mailboxes. This new acquaintance knew little of me beyond the simple recognition that we were neighbors. We were around the same height, Lisa a little heavier, and I a bit older. Both of us had salon-colored hair; hers was sandy blonde, while mine was dark brunette. Both of us wore well-used warm jackets and old blue jeans. My jeans were decorated with swipes of paint and caulk from years of projects. Some blotches were new.

"It's cold out here," Lisa said, pantomiming an exaggerated shiver.

I wasn't sure if she was speaking to herself or to me, so I nodded in agreement as I sifted through junk mail.

Lisa took a step closer and asked, "How are you doing in that house?"

I moved into this neighborhood four weeks ago, nineteen months after Jack passed away. In my old neighborhood, I lived next to people I'd known for twenty years.

"Oh, I'm doing okay," I stammered.

I eliminated "Fine" as a response months ago. People loved to ask a widow, *How are you doing?* and the truth was I wasn't fine, but hanging on, some days better than others. Just "Okay."

"The house needs a lot of work," I said. Not knowing Lisa's relationship with the previous owner, not wanting to offend, I added quickly, "…to make it mine."

I kept it together in front of my new neighbor, but a chill ran up my spine as we talked. Lisa didn't know about Jack, and one doesn't typically blurt out, "I'm a widow," in an initial conversation.

When she asked about the house, I stifled a groan. The changes I was making, would Lisa pass judgment, decide I was doing too much or too little, and tell others? Did she know the state of disrepair inside? The kitchen oven had crusted black walls and racks, even after two self-cleaning cycles, and the burnt spills and scratches on the glass range left me one option: replacement. The microwave had a broken turnstile. Previous owners removed shelving and speakers from walls and ceilings in several rooms, which left numerous holes to be filled and textured before painting, a skill I had because Jack taught me how.

I said nothing to Lisa of the hours I'd spent putting down the royal blue painter's tape on molding and ceiling vents, removing outlet covers, and painting both the primer and the paint over what I called "baby-poo-poo yellow," a shade of German mustard that covered almost every wall. Even the exterior vinyl siding of this two-story house was this awful, dirty yellow; the white trim on windows and peaks did little to distract from the "poop" appearance. The main floor half-bath, the upstairs second bath, and the laundry room were in-gasp-dark battleship gray. Worst yet were the two children's rooms upstairs: one chartreuse green and the other royal blue, including the ceilings and closets, all of which eventually needed two coats of primer and two coats of cream. Every damn wall in those bright green and "battleship gray" rooms had four coats of time and effort.

I still lived around unpacked boxes, pushed to the middle of rooms for a whole month while I painted each wall my neutral cream color. I didn't have the mental energy to pick decorative tones for each room. One color was simple, once I'd chosen it from the dozen shades of white, which wasn't simple. Besides, I lacked an artistic eye. A voice in my head warned, whenever I brought home another paint store brochure of complementary hues, *Don't buy an arty color. You'll end up hating it in a month and repainting that wall back to a neutral color.*

"I'm doing okay," I told Lisa. But in this new house, every cell of my body screamed, *I miss you, Jackson, and our lives we once had.*

I needed his hands to lift boxes, and his height to paint the high corners of the staircase and ceilings. I wanted his second opinion. Jack was my sympathetic listener, my encourager, the person I needed when I was slumped on a stair, overwhelmed, and tired. I missed *our* old neighborhood, the friends who checked on me after Jack's death. Instead, I was alone.

But our old three-story house was too big for me and filled with too many shadows. Staying there would have only burrowed me into the past. I knew each step I took would result in droplets of courage, determination, and strength into my soul's large bucket. The grief would ease.

Sorting through the mail at this new address, I missed Jack's help. We used to make teamwork of it: open the envelopes, toss the ads into the recycle bin, and groan (or argue) together at the credit card bill. I craved the letters addressed to "Tally and Jack Reynolds," proof that we were once a couple, or to "Jack Reynolds," proof that he was once alive. Fewer and fewer for him came with each passing month. I hugged them to my heart when they did and whispered, *You found me, Bubba.*

But each envelope sent to Jack meant a sad chore for me. Did neighbors ever wonder what I mumbled out to the sky?

"Hey, Jackson, Red Cross wants you to donate. How much do you want the check to be? … Sorry, Bubba, I must tell them that I will take care of it from now on."

But what I missed most was daily, simple, face-to-face conversation. The only person I spoke to regularly was the paint store clerk. Though I was unsure how to respond, my heart felt warmed by Lisa's question. Someone knew I was alive inside that house.

"You got a deal on the house," Lisa said. "Kath told us that you bickered down the price of the place. They had no option but to accept your offer. You knew they were heading into bankruptcy, right?"

I turned my gaze to the cedar trees over her shoulders, watched a crow fly by, and said, "Hmm. No, I didn't know about the bankruptcy. How sad for them that the housing market crashed."

Could she see the fury that rose red into my cheeks? I didn't want to disclose the details of the negotiations or discuss the final price of my new home with a stranger. I clamped my jaws together to keep myself from hissing. *Well, they frickin' lied to you. There were brand-new homes down the street that I could have had for a cheaper price.* That sounded combative, and that wasn't how I wanted to be. After all, she heard only one side.

Months ago, when I found this house, I resolved that the energy surrounding this home purchase would be kind and soft: no drawn-out negotiations, no bitterness from either side. I was willing to compromise, be flexible. I had grown sharp and hard edges from the loss of Jack, a quick temper, and sullen moods. But I was sparring enough with the heavens, asking, *Why him? Why me? Why now?* I didn't have it in me to make this process a fight.

I needed a house where I wouldn't see Jack in the walls and tiles, light fixtures, or paint swatches we debated together. I needed a place in which he never walked. I wanted to plant my own roots, literally. I craved new soil under my nails, a garden that would bring the joy of late-winter purple crocuses, spring red and yellow tulips, white pansies, and summer lilacs. And once I settled in, a new dog was at the top of my list. Seven months was the longest I had gone without a dog, and the little rescued critter would need space in this new home to play.

My real estate agent chatted with the seller, Kath, a thin, thirty-something blonde with the tired eyes of a mom with two boys under five. They sat at her kitchen table and reviewed the "comps," those houses of similar size and value in the area, including the new construction a quarter mile away. Public records showed the couple bought high and lost their large down payment in the nose-diving market, and now the house had been on the market for half a year.

My agent urged Kath, "You will not get your asking price in this market. And you have a serious buyer."

In just a few days, the deal was done with a four-step dance: my offer, their counter, my counter, their acceptance. Gentle and generous and fair.

Although the closing was on a Wednesday in early December, I let the sellers stay until Saturday to make it easier on the working couple with two little ones. Kath and her husband, Paul, agreed that I could bring in some of my items, line them along one wall in the garage on closing day, and start my big move-in on Sunday. Pre-dawn

Wednesday, I drove the first of two five-hour round trips to the cabin, loaded up what was stored in its garage, and returned to my new house.

As I drove Jack's loaded white truck down the driveway, around their large U-Haul truck, I saw what neighbors saw when the garage door was opened: the entire space was stacked head-high and wall-to-wall with camping gear, reminding me of the insides of a large Goodwill trailer of discarded items. No space for me along the wall. I sought out Paul, a handsome thirty-something man in work jeans, gathering garden tools at the side of the house. He apologized, and with the help of his friend, a young, slender man with a mop of curly hair, we moved their things inward.

Once Paul returned to the side yard, his friend, whose first name I never caught, passed me while I unloaded my truck. He shook his head and grimaced.

"I think you're mean to make them leave so soon," he snipped at me.

That word "*mean*" slapped. Apparently, Kath and Paul hadn't told their friends about my generosity. They stayed four days rent-free after the closing. Although the signed contract stated that all appliances were to remain, I gave them the washer and dryer, thinking it would be heartless to take those from a family with two small boys; I would find a local laundromat or wash items in the sink until I bought new ones. Was anyone told that I waived the inspector's four-page report? They didn't have the money, so it would have been cruel of me to push for repairs. All I needed was a three-foot corridor of space along one wall of the garage that Wednesday.

Keep it simple. Be gentle. Be kind.

On the other hand, I addressed all but one item on the inspector's report for my home, Jack's and mine, because, after all, the buyer was a widow, too. My buyer requested only ten of the twenty issues on the two-page report, but I wanted to hand over the house in good shape. I skipped only one task on the list because I ran out of time: new hand railings outside and in, caulking around newly installed windows, a new door lock, insulation of crawl space, piping to exterior for water heater, and others. I even replaced the used washing machine with a new one. I left a beautiful house for her because I knew what it took to live alone.

Be fair. Stay peaceful.

I needed rest and calm for my heart. The prep, selling, packing, and moving had been taxing. I had lost several pounds, my appetite was gone, and I had dark half-moons under my eyes from sixteen-hour workdays and irregular sleep. I felt fragile, fearing that the first virus that flew by would land me in bed for a week. I was never far from crying.

I wanted to stand in the driveway of my new house and have a joyful moment. I wanted to shout, *You're all mine. I will take good care of you. I promise!* Instead, I stood blinking in surprise at the stranger who had just called me "mean" for needing to take up a bit of space.

"This house is *legally* mine *today*," I shot back at the helper with a hot stare, the one I gave to misbehaving students that froze them in their tracks. His face reddened, and his steps clanged on the metal ramp as he retreated into the U-Haul. He never looked back.

I sought out Paul by the side of the house, kneeling at a pile of dirt. I stomped up to him, the word still souring in my head.

"What the fuck, Paul? What's with your friend saying I was being 'mean' to make you move out now? The house is legally mine today."

His mouth opened in surprise. Standing up, he rested the shovel against his chest and said, "I am so sorry. My friend is a little slow," pointing to his head. "He doesn't always get what is going on. I'll talk to him."

Suddenly, I could see it, Paul, too, was so tired. I could almost hear his thinking, *Please, not one more problem.* Poor man. After seeing the insides of the garage, I could only imagine the insides of the house. This couple was on overload. They'd be lucky to get out in a week.

Besides, I knew better than to react the way I had. I'd worked with many developmentally disabled students over my years in the schools, but had totally overlooked his friend's slow or non-responses to my comments when we were clearing space in the garage. I thought he hadn't heard or was ignoring me completely.

"Sure lucky to have no rain, uh?" I'd asked him.

"…Yeah."

"Are you a friend of Kath's or Paul's?"

Silence.

"You know what they say about people who help others move: must have a strong back, but a weak mind."

He'd turned away. Not even a smile.

How did I get so combative, so quickly, with Paul? I could have inquired about a possible misunderstanding, but no, I threw my anger at someone who was equally stressed, overworked, and fatigued. I knew I should apologize.

What sort of person am I becoming? Help me, Jackson. God, help me.

That weekend, I felt my new neighbors watching from their windows, saw them walking by and turning to stare at the orange and white twenty-foot U-Haul truck, white Ford one-ton truck, and two twenty-something men helping a fifty-something woman move in. I waved at them when our eyes met, but saw that most hands remained at their sides and heads snapped forward, as if embarrassed for being curious. What would it take to wave back to a new neighbor? Had they heard false stories of the sale?

I wondered what they were thinking. Probably assuming that these young men were my sons. Perhaps they thought unkindly, *That's all the help she's got?* Or noticed, *She's got more rooms than furniture.* It took two trips for the two men to carry in a large, thick glass tabletop and then back to the U-Haul for its thick, blackish metal frame base. Another trip for the treadmill, and back for the queen mattress and bedframe in pieces. One of the men bear-hugged the sole large garment box into the house. *Only one?* Boxes and boxes and boxes went inside and filled the garage. *What, no washer and dryer? No dresser or side tables, or book cabinets? A four-drawer file cabinet, but not a desk? No couch or chairs? What about a TV?* Just a couple of tall reading lamps. *Tsk, how barren it will be in there.* It only took ninety minutes to empty both trucks and lower the garage door.

In that moment, I deeply missed the old neighborhood. Those neighbors would have come down and helped, brought snacks and beers. Women would have offered to clean the inside of cabinets, pantries, and closets, and then unpack items into them. They would stop to share memories of Jack with me. Someone would have ordered pizza for when we were done, and we'd sit on the floor amidst the boxes to eat, drink, and laugh.

Here, I was only that "mean" woman who bought Kath and Paul's house. *Oh, Jackson, should I have stayed put in our home?*

Thank God I asked my stepson Steven, and Josh the son of a dear friend, to put the bed together before they left on moving day. The bed was from the basement guest room of the old house, where Jack and I slept a couple of nights a year when the hottest summer days made our lofted bedroom unbearable. The guest room was where I occasionally escaped from Jack's snoring. After the house was staged, I slept there. Dragging that mattress up to the "mistress's bedroom" in this new house and assembling the pine frame alone would have pushed me into tears. I was so tired, arms stretched by all the lifting, legs heavy with the repeated fourteen-stair climb to the second floor and back down.

I will eventually paint what will be the new guest room, move this old guest bed there, and buy a new bed set for myself. Later.

The U-Haul was gone by midday, and I returned in Jack's truck. Eventually, my maroon and silver Subaru Baja, which often got me pegged as a WSU Cougar fan, was parked in the driveway. Two vehicles. Did the neighbors wonder when the second driver would appear?

Aside from the sounds of cardboard being tossed into the garage, screws being drilled, and nails being pounded, no one saw or heard much of me as I settled into the new place. I ventured into the wintry, wet cold to put up a couple of strings of holiday lights on the eaves. In the kitchen window, I set up two four-foot plastic trees atop TV tables, and they twinkled with colorful lights. Although it was hard to find that sense of joy within me on my second holiday alone, the house said, *Happy Holidays.*

Soon, I'd filled the truck for a Goodwill run, and things moved hastily from the old to the new place for no other reason than sentimentality or pure exhaustion. I loaded up the oak cabinet, which once held Jack's LP records and cassette tape collection, his old stereo equipment, and a couple of large speakers. More of his possessions, gone.

In the present moment, a plethora of boxes, large and small, old wine boxes from Trader Joe's, new boxes from the moving company, all well-marked with a wide black marker, filled rooms and rooms like giant tan building blocks. Whenever I passed by the five-foot-tall garment box of Jack's dress clothes, which towered over the others in the main room, I patted on its heavily taped top and said, "Hey, Jackson. Quite a mess, uh?" or "What do you think, Bud?"

I rearranged boxes to create narrow paths that serpentined through the garage, into the kitchen, down the hall to the family room, and snaked their way into the upstairs rooms. It was a dance of side steps, step overs, and occasional bumps and stumbles to the floor. I craved a straight line. I wanted order.

"If you need help, call us," offered my Friday morning coffee friends, Denise, Sandy, and Joyce. They were former colleagues, at one time in the same school, but now scattered: Denise remained in the same school and handled ASB business in the front office, Sandy was at the alternative high school, and Joyce taught Spanish at two different junior highs. They all knew Jack, were all lifetime friends living in the area, who cared enough to stop by after work for a brief visit. But my friends were drained from their own busy lives, days full of students, staff, and parents. They came, and they left to spouses who were alive and awaiting their return.

My priority was cleaning, shelves, cabinets, and drawers that should hold only *my* dirt and dust from now on. A friend whom I'd met through the PTA at my old school came by and tackled the dirty fingerprints and food residues on the interior and exterior of the kitchen cabinets. A soccer teammate with a housecleaning business brought her daughter by, and they spent hours scrubbing both bathrooms, upstairs and down. The glass shower stall was opaque with soap scum, and the two sets of sinks, mirrors, and countertops were spattered with water residue, toothpaste dots, and grime. Toilets hadn't been scrubbed in weeks. The acrid smell of old urine rose from the vinyl floor; Kath and Paul had a five-year-old still working on his aim.

I scoured the stainless-steel kitchen sink and the dark green speckled granite countertops. I unpacked cookware and a few cans of food onto the pantry floor and got those empty boxes tossed into the garage. The pantry needed work: the wood shelves needed glue-down shelf paper to hide permanent food stains, and the walls and ceiling needed new paint. More jobs for later.

So much for waving off the inspection report, I thought bitterly. I had saved the financially desperate family hours of cleaning, repairs, and replacements. As I scrubbed and scrubbed, I felt used. But when my angry voice spiked, *Damn them!* I stopped myself.

Breathe in peace. Don't bring anger into this home. Breathe.

As a rule, painting walls came before unpacking boxes. An "I-love-to-paint" friend offered help. Getting out of her car, she proudly held up her favorite painting tool, a four-inch roller. I stopped myself from muttering within earshot, *Ya gotta be kidding me?* Help was help, even if it was only four inches at a time. I prepped and hand-brushed all corners and edges of what became my study, and my standard ten-inch roller did two of the largest walls and the cove entry of the room to her two smaller walls.

I refused my friends' offers to help with the unpacking. I needed to razor open the boxes and unpack each item alone, feel its weight in my hand, let my fingers glide over edges and curves, relive the story within. I needed time to find the right place in this new house for each of our old things, to make this place mine.

My body was so worn from the physical work of moving in; when unexpected grief slipped around my ribs and squeezed, my knees buckled. I would rock and chant, *I miss you, I miss you so much, Jackson,* on the tan shag carpet, on the thin dark cherry laminate floor of the kitchen, on the cement floor of the garage. Each time I crumbled, I'd dry my eyes with a T-shirt sleeve and attempt to place memories back on a mental shelf.

Focus, focus, focus.

Finish, finish, finish.

When I called about house insurance, I was told that my rate would go up in the new neighborhood, a "higher crime incident area of town," the agent said. My heart raced as I processed this. I picked a house without much research.

Am I safe here?

Forgetting to give me the code to open the garage door when they left, Paul left a phone message with the numbers days later. I missed Jack as I stood in the cold of a rainy morning: I would have read the instructions while Jack punched in our new numbers. I failed over and over to reset the code. Spewing swear words and crying, I gave up, taking out the battery so no one could use the old code to break into the house.

Jack and I had always shared a spare key with a neighbor and hid another outside. Should I do that here? Should I be afraid of the surrounding homes with clear views of the front of my house? What if someone discovers my hiding place? What if the driver of a passing car sees me lift a flowerpot on the porch and enter my house? Would the key be safer with a neighbor than in the yard somewhere?

With a chuckle, Lisa handed me the house key as I stood on her front porch for the second time in one week, asking for the spare. "Your poor brain," she said.

I had locked myself out yet again. The doorknob lock position was the opposite of the old house: what was "unlocked" there was "locked" here.

"I think it's sort of brave that you gave us a house key. You didn't even know us when you handed it over," Lisa said.

"Just a good gut feeling," I said, and smiled.

A few weeks later, another neighbor called the police because I left the front door completely open when I drove off to the cabin for a few days. The police entered, checked for damage, and locked the door on their way out. It turned out I wasn't alone here. I had thoughtful new neighbors.

Thanks, Bud. Ya did well in helping me.

I was a post-menopausal widow who feared that I was in over my head with all that a house entailed: the maintenance, the expenses, the home security. Maybe a condo would have been a better idea, as friends suggested, a smaller turn-key place. But I needed the dirt of a garden and wasn't ready to share my walls with other people. I imagined my new neighbors watching over me as I lost a bit of my sanity each day. Would they eventually see drawn curtains and newspapers piled up on the driveway, hear the yapping of pent-up dogs, and remark to each other, *"Old Lady Reynolds lost another screw?"* Would they send someone for a welfare check?

"Living alone?" Lisa asked as we lingered at the mailboxes. She must have noticed that no one else came out of the house or retrieved the mail.

Turning my eyes downward to the ground, I didn't want to see her reaction when I said, "My husband passed away seventeen months ago."

The number of months slipped easily from my lips, no need for a mental calculation. I still knew to the day, and, if I stopped and thought, to the hour.

I paused and added, "Cancer, skin cancer," to answer her unasked question. I swallowed the grief that was gathering in my throat and behind my eyes.

"I am sorry to hear that," Lisa said. Nothing more. She had no Jack stories to share.

Whenever I had conversations with anyone in this new neighborhood, I floundered. How much should I share of my past? Should I point out that the watercolor print or the metal art we bought down in Cannon Beach and reveal my history with Jack? Or should I avoid bringing the past in, let the neighbors see me as a single woman, keep the conversation on the new wall colors, the unpacking, and future landscaping plans?

I often slipped on icy pronouns when I talked to people. My house, my things, but that was his white truck in the driveway. When I intentionally picked words that removed Jack from the conversation, "*My truck needs new tabs,*" the words tasted like sour milk but saved me from having to explain.

Unless I slipped.

Coming back from a jog one afternoon, I met Lisa out in her driveway talking with a woman I didn't know. I stopped and chatted with them for a moment, and then said, "See you, ladies. Need to change my clothes and take Jack's truck to get a load of soil."

I felt the air thicken between us when I said Jack's name. Lisa's friend raised her eyebrows.

"I thought you were a widow," she said, like a parent who caught a teenager in a lie.

I stammered, "I am, and that was his truck. I gotta go."

I didn't want to explain the details. Lisa would probably fill her in. I turned, went down my driveway, and felt the heat of my life being discussed behind my back.

The box that was marked "FRAGILE, JACK" on all five sides, underlined twice, contained items swaddled in bubble wrap. The ceramic eight-inch white and turquoise dog in a "Let's play" stance was a gift. I bought it at the beach one summer behind Jack's back and sneaked it home in my luggage to hide it away until Christmas. That dog had lived for years on a shelf in Jack's study. I placed it atop my newly purchased hutch in my newly painted study so that it could watch over me.

The wood-framed certificates, honoring Jack's service to state and national high school activities and wrestling officials' associations, just didn't belong on the walls of the new house. *What do I do with them, Jack?* The box was placed in a closet to deal with later.

In my haste to pack the old house as quickly as possible, I'd thrown everything from Jack's bedstand into a box: unread paperback spy novels, a Bible, a wrestling rules book, the emails from friends I printed and read to him while he was bedridden, and old birthday cards. The box remained sealed in the new house, tucked next to the box of certificates.

Then there was a box of soft sentimental material: commercially embroidered patches cut from his polo shirts, one of his black-and-white striped referee shirts, and cloth for the backside of a winter day project that I thought of as "Jack's quilt." That box got pushed under a shelf in the laundry room.

Meanwhile, the five-foot-tall garment box stood above the other boxes in the middle of the family room. Inside were Jack's dress shirts, shoes, and suits. The clothes were wrapped in garment bags, each encased in another thick black garbage bag, and silver duct tape sealed the gap around the top of the hangers. Three or four straps of duct tape sealed any open edges of the box. At the bottom of the box were his black brogues. He'd only worn them once, the night we attended "*The Phantom of the Opera,*" his favorite musical, on Broadway. Since that trip to New York was one week after his last radiation treatment for the cancer that had traveled to his brain, we took a taxi to and from the theater, even though it was only four blocks away from our hotel. That was his last birthday adventure, six weeks before his last heartbeat. The soles of those shoes were still smooth.

I knew the smells that those clothes held: the sweetness of the Royall Lyme aftershave, the earthiness of sweat, his freshly bathed skin. In the early months after he passed, the rawness of loss drove me to find him in the only place I could, which was in his clothes. In his closet, I could relive the comfort of burying my face into his neck, inhaling deeply. I could feel my arms circle around his neck, his arms pulling me tight into him. The tickle of his lips on my neck, the dance of our tongues, the arousal that ran up from our hips. I could hear Jack tell me, "Nice ass," as we undressed.

Now I felt his love reach out from the garment box, a warmth that circled around me. Unpacking that box was for much later.

As the months passed, I saw Lisa's friends come to visit her, women from around the neighborhood coming and going from her front door as I drove off on errands. Often, I thought I saw heads turn toward my house from her porch, or a pair of eyes scrutinizing out from her front window. I imagined them asking, *Have you seen much of her?*

I imagined Lisa's reply, too. *No, not much. Although she sure is bringing in gallons of paint, and early in the mornings, too. For hours yesterday, I heard hammering and the squeal of a screw gun echoing from the garage. When the garage door was up, I saw that she'd dismantled all those shelves Paul built in there. Wouldn't that bust his gut to see his work undone? An appliance store truck arrived a while back, and two men brought in a washer, dryer, microwave, range, and refrigerator. A bit later, a furniture store truck showed up and brought in a bed, nightstands, and a couch. And then, as if that wasn't enough, the Geek Squad came and set up a TV. Aren't you curious what she's done to the insides of Kath and Paul's house?*

Inside the house, inside my reality, I remained focused on unpacking, painting, and buying furniture. I left windows open to diffuse the smell of fresh paint and bleach. The recently delivered three-piece navy-blue sectional couch demanded that I clear all boxes out of the family room.

"Gotta move you upstairs, Bud," I said to the garment box.

I pushed the box down the hall from the family room, rocked it up fourteen steps one at a time, and leaned it gently inside the walk-in closet next to the bathroom. After a trip to the hardware store that afternoon, I tapped the box.

"Gotta move ya again, Jackson." I rocked the box back out into the bathroom. I needed room to maneuver in Jack's half of the closet. I set to work installing new shelves and rods for his shirts, jackets, and the dress clothes from the garment box, then stepped back to survey my work. With the shelving in place, I returned to the tall garment box.

"It's time, Jack." My heart raced. A quiver ran down my arm as I gripped the knife: time to open the box and hang his dress clothes so I could come visit him here.

I made so many careful slashes into so many layers of silver tape. As I finally unfolded the lid, *Oh God, no, no!* The wet cement musk of the storage unit overwhelmed me. Rising like smoke, the unpleasant smell had permeated the cardboard.

No, no, no!

But surely, I thought, the two layers of plastic had protected the clothes. I grabbed one of the three sets of hangers, choosing the bag that held three dress shirts from amongst the others, the black dress suit, the new sports plaid jacket, and the khaki pants on heavy wood hangers from Men's Warehouse. Cutting the duct tape that sealed the black bags to the top of hangers, I let the tape and bag fall to the bottom of the box, lifted out the garment bag, and laid it flat on the floor of the bathroom.

Oh, please still be there.

Slowly, I unzipped the garment bag and peered inside to see the pastel blue, white, and cream dress shirts. My heartbeat quickened; my mouth went dry.

Please, God, please.

With a shaking hand, I lifted out the blue shirt, still crisply pressed. I slowly pulled the fine cotton to my nose. With eyes closed, I took a long inhale.

Jack didn't come to the new house.

Chapter 18
[Poem]

Losing Me

I am like the invisible man

who watches his body cells disappear:

his hands, limbs, and face

become transparent until

finally, there is nothing left

but his voice. I am losing

what makes me unique, distinct

from everything around me.

Chameleon-like, I meld into

the surrounding landscape,

blend into walls, disappear

amidst crowds. I don't know

who I am anymore.

Chapter 19
Show Up: Therapist and Another Widow's Advice

"How did you survive those early days, after Jerry passed?"

My friendship with Lou Ann started four years ago in a support group for the widowed. Her husband had died from an unexpected heart attack. She was a few years younger and a few pounds heavier than I was, and we both wore smiles that contrasted with our painful pasts. We sat for lunch in a local Vietnamese restaurant Lou Ann loved, with its red fabric walls, black chopsticks on ivory linen tables, and the scent of garlic in the air. The food was perfect, and so was the company, neither of us liked to eat out alone. I wanted to hear from Lou Ann that I wasn't the only one whose life was turned upside down by widowhood. And yet she'd survived. *How did she do it?*

Lou Ann stopped chewing her food and leaned over her entrée. Her blue eyes peered through her dark, wide-rimmed glasses as she arched one brow. Her auburn hair, cut in a neat bob, draped over her face.

"I just... *did*," Lou Ann snapped, as if she were teaching a small child simple math. "How else? You just survive it." She eyed her plate and finished chewing. The simplicity of her words stung. And yet, I understood.

"Because nothing happens waiting for Jack to walk up the porch steps and enter the front door?" During those early months, I spent hours watching out the window, my mind frozen in icy denial.

"Nope. And nothing happens languishing in bed," she countered. Taking another bite, she pointed her empty fork at me and added, "Or in a vodka bottle."

Lou Ann drank through that first year with Jerry gone, playing continuous games of computer solitaire, gaining weight. I lost pounds eating popcorn for dinner, occasionally drank too much red wine, broke down into tears as soon as the shower water hit me, and frequently collapsed in front of the stereo speaker, hearing the opening notes of a love song, doubling the pain by tapping "repeat." I lost minutes, hours, even days, without a clue of how I'd spent the time. *How did other widows survive? Was I normal? What is "normal" in this new widowhood hell?*

After Jack died, I returned to my therapist, Kate. She had guided my healing from a chaotic childhood with dysfunctional parents, issues that had snuck into my adulthood. I saw her immediately after the diagnosis, the day before his first of many biopsy surgeries, and again after his death. I arrived on time for those appointments, unlike most social gatherings, when I either arrived late or totally forgot.

The pain of grief was a thousand pinpricks, all day and night. I pleaded with both my God and my therapist in the first year after Jack's death. "Tell me what to do, how to survive this, and I will do it."

Grief groups and workshops? Sign me up.

Read more on healing? Give me titles to buy, although I had neither the concentration nor comprehension for anything longer than one or two pages.

Journal more? Tell me how many pages to write each day, although my words often jumbled in my mind, and the pen felt heavy in my hand.

Kate had the look of a French aristocrat, with petite, fine facial features. She was an educated woman whose words had purpose, clarity, and sincerity. But she gave off no aristocratic vibes in her office; she was Montanan, grounded in the earth, deeply spiritual, and a survivor of cancer, which all melded into her wisdom and compassion.

In the soft lighting of Kate's office, nestled on one of the two apricot-colored couches, was Honey, her therapy dog. Honey was a tan Wheaton terrier who always greeted me with tail wags, doggie kisses, and waited for the treats I carried in my jacket pocket.

"I'm glad you're here," she greeted me with a hug. In my sessions, I typically sat with Honey on the floor, but today I sank onto the other couch. Kate rolled her desk chair to face me and, looking into my eyes, asked, "How are you doing?"

Immediately, my eyes moistened. Kate listened to my words and, as always, remained present through the occasional silences that stretched between us. Several times during the session, she added an insight or redirected my thinking.

"Tally, have you thought about…?"

"Did I hear you right when you said…?"

Suffice it to say, I trusted Kate. But when we reached the end of our hour, she offered me the words, "Show up." I felt like she was handing me a useless bit of fortune cookie advice.

Say what?

I felt defensive, then combative, like I'd done something wrong. *I got out of bed, got clothes on, and showed up on time here. Didn't I? I* kept those retorts in my head but felt them in my fists. Was my therapist really offering me these two words for survival? So tidy, so compact, so easy to toss around, like an airplane seat cushion that was supposed to save me from drowning while I was flying over jagged mountains.

As the hour hand of the clock signaled the end of the therapy session, Kate wrote four phrases on a yellow Post-it note:

SHOW UP.

PAY ATTENTION.

TELL YOUR TRUTH WITHOUT SHAME OR JUDGMENT.

BE OPEN TO THE OUTCOME.

With a hug, she said, "See you next week."

At home, I taped Kate's note to the inside of the cabinet where I stored my morning teas and cups, but rarely looked at it again. Most of these phrases demanded more thinking power than I had available. But those two words, *Show up*, stayed with me.

With a snort, Lou Ann replied, "Hmph. My shrink said things like that, too. I just pretended I understood so he wouldn't go on and on."

We both laughed, and how good that felt. Grief bottled up my laughter for so long; I could only smile, maybe give a soft chuckle. My friends tried to arouse my Irish wit, but nothing was funny. This laughter was fresh and cool, like stepping outside after a new snowfall for a breath.

Recalling those early months, I felt my shoulders droop. "I hurt every time I stepped out of the house alone, and I hurt inside the house without Jack. Why go anywhere or try anything?"

Pinching her thumb and index finger together, then pulling them apart slightly so that only a sliver of light shone through, Lou Ann explained, "But I bet it hurt *that* much less each time you 'showed up,' as your therapist said. And that's why we did it. That tiny amount was still better than nothing."

Yes, Lou Ann was like me. She understood that healing was a long, long road with very, very small steps. Some steps went backward. Some forward. Others were back-and-forth-and-back-and-forth until the wobbling finally stopped.

The first winter holidays without Jack fell a mere five months after his death. So early in my pain, this season full of tradition, family, and romance, first Thanksgiving pie without Jack, first Christmas party as a widow. I bruised and bled as I rammed into each "first."

My non-widowed friends were alarmed. "Slow down, Tally," one friend admonished. "You don't have to do everything this first year."

Tell me when, I yelled in my head. *When will it not hurt? What will make it easier to be the new single among a world of pairs? When?*

I felt like a swimmer at the edge of an unheated pool on a winter day. Friends advised me to enter the frigid water by taking the steps, one by one, a gradual immersion. Instead, I jumped in, for no other reason than to get the shock over with as quickly as possible. Each headfirst dive stung me to my core and splashed up waves of grief.

I ate Thanksgiving dinner at one friend's table, Christmas brunch at another, and Christmas dinner at yet a third, passed like a bucket of water in a fire brigade from one hostess to the next. I was too proud to show up at these parties with Tupperware containers in hand, even though my own kitchen was empty. Even though my friends would have eagerly filled them up and felt grateful they could do something, anything, to help me. But I couldn't ask for what I needed during those early days.

When I left the homes of my generous friends, I was met with silence, silence inside the car, stillness in the house where Annie B, with a tail wave, greeted me if she was awake, and a clean kitchen without any aroma of baked holiday dishes. There was no conversation floating between the washer of dirty pans and the drier. No soft hand on my back, no kiss on my cheek. No teamwork: *While you finish up, I'll take Annie B for a walk.*

But I did my best to show up.

My inner child wanted all the Christmas holiday traditions for my first year of widowhood: angels, reindeer, snowmen, and Santa figurines scattered on flat surfaces around the house. I wanted multi-colored lights on the outside of the house, and the smell of a decorated evergreen tree to greet me each time I walked onto the main floor. But each item I took out of the holiday decoration boxes was heavier than the last. The stockings were labeled with our names, "Jack," "Tally," and "Annie B," each with a special hook for displaying on the mantel. I ran my hand over the soft red boot and white-furred top with "Jack" in silver glittered glue. Peering inside, I saw flashes of the prior year's Christmas preparations, when I sat at the dining room table to pore over holiday advertisements and wandered store aisles to find the "perfect" gifts for a man who might become bedridden in the months ahead. I remember thinking, knowing, it might be his last Christmas.

Damn me for being right.

This year's dilemma: To hang Jack's stocking or not? To stay in the past, or live on?

Get this frickin' Christmas over with, I yelled silently at myself. *Hang the damn stockings!*

Joy withered.

I bought my first tree without Jack at a local drugstore. There was a row of small, rejected trees leaning in their wood stands, or still in webbing, against the side of the building. They appeared like the sad dogs at the pound begging to be taken home. I brought an unwrapped six-footer, placed it in the back of Jack's truck, and tied it securely down. At home, I cut off the last three inches of the trunk and placed it in a bucket of warm water in the garage, like Jack always did. Pitch stuck to my hands, and I didn't know how to get it off.

Tell me, Jack, what to do?

The next day, I got the tree inside and placed it into the base. After numerous attempts to get the crooked trunk as straight as possible, adjust bolts, step back, evaluate, curse, repeat steps, I placed the red tree blanket around it. My lungs filled with the sweet pine scent, and my inner child smiled.

But I hit a wall when I reached for the ornament box. Jack relished the placement of each ornament, humming holiday songs as he went. *Ah, his smile.* I always hung the lights outside, because I was surer-footed on the ladder and more comfortable with heights. Over the years, as we bought a new ornament every Christmas, I started penning the purchase date on the back of each one. Opening the box, I pulled out a Santa wearing a tool belt bought during a major remodel, a little boy wrapped in winter wear with poles and skis from when we skied all over the Pacific Northwest, and a dog holding a bone from the year when we got Annie B. This was like flipping the pages of a photo album.

Do you remember when we went to Whistler, and it was raining?

Which student made this cute ornament of you?

Without the answers, my questions fell like dried needles onto the floor. I walked away from the unadorned tree.

Days later, sniffling on Kate's couch with my arms extended out as if pleading for alms, I asked, "What do I do? I can't decorate the tree, it was Jack's job, and, what's worse, there are no gifts underneath it."

"Oh, Tally," Kate nudged, "Ask for help. Surely a neighbor will decorate it, and your friends will get you something."

I tallied the toll of reciprocal gifts: the drive to a mall with its packed parking lot, the walk down crowded aisles, the long check-out lines, wrapping the presents at home, and, finally, gift delivery. I sank deeper into the couch cushion. Finding that kind of energy, both mental and physical, was like trying to squeeze a drop of water out of a dry sponge.

"Ask for help," she reminded me again. "Your friends would love a chance to be there for you as you face this first Christmas." With a smirk, as if she read my mind, Kate added, "Even *without* getting a gift from you."

What I wanted for the holidays was simple, but not found in stores: a reminder to breathe, more than a few hours of sleep at a time, and a break from the unexpected bouts of crying. My friends couldn't wrap those up for me.

But I made a weak promise. "Yes, I will ask for help, Kate."

Upon arriving home, I trudged up the street to a neighbor's home. *Get it over with before this idea seems stupid.*

Janet and Deborah were twin sisters, neighbors, and reliable friends; they'd come to my aid when Jack was dying. Avid gardener that I was, I had no energy to deal with the fallen or still-hanging brown camellia blossoms by the garage, and I grimaced at them every time I walked by with Annie B. Within an hour of posting the need for a gardener on my blog, Janet and Deborah came to my rescue. They were good souls.

Jack could never tell these women apart like I could; after an encounter, he'd tell me he ran into "one of the twins," or ask me later, "Which one was that?" I knew that Janet had a rounder face, Deborah was slightly taller, and both had dark hair, but in different styles. I could even hear the difference in their voices.

I knocked on the dark wood door and prayed no one was there so I could return home and say at my next session, *Yes, I tried, Kate.* After all, we didn't specify how many times I had to ask. I wanted the tree done, but with Jack's passing, everything seemed harder, more difficult, more complex, more taxing. I wanted easy. I wished I could telepathically relay my needs. That's all the energy I had, but given the state of my brain, even those ESP messages would probably arrive garbled.

Deborah opened the door. Her brown eyes widened in surprise at my presence, and she crooned softly, "Tally." She pulled me into her chest as my tears fell. A floral smell radiated from her sweatshirt as she held me tight.

"We miss him, too," she whispered in my ear. After a few moments, I leaned back, and she let go. Both of us pulled out tissues from our pockets and wiped our eyes and noses.

"Come on in. What can we do for you?"

Inside their stone entry, I stuttered, "I need help," and explained both the tree decoration job and the request for gifts. I tried to ignore the part of me that translated *I need help* to *I am too weak/stupid/incapable without Jack.*

"Jan-Jan and I would love to," Deborah smiled as she volunteered her sister away at work. "When do you want it done?"

"Is it possible tomorrow afternoon? I have theatre tickets and the house will be empty from noon 'til around five, except for Annie B."

Oh, God, it's always empty except for the dog. My eyes refilled.

"Get me a house key and we'll get it done. Anything else?" she added.

I calculated quickly: I would have to walk the twenty yards to home to retrieve the key, then another twenty yards back to Deborah, and then another twenty yards back to home. Sixty long damn yards that felt like miles, another knock, another conversation at the door.

"How about I just leave it under the doormat?"

"No problem," she said with a smile.

Bless you, dear neighbor.

More hugs. More tissues.

My brain began a bank ledger. How could I ever repay them for their help? I struggled with anything that felt one-sided, how much harder it was to receive than give. This was a familiar feeling; after knee surgery years ago, during a week of rides offered by a generous colleague, she grew impatient with me thanking her excessively, insisting, "I owe you, Shar," every morning and afternoon.

"Damn it, Tally," Shar barked one morning, "let me have my feel-good moment and enjoy being here for you. You're not the only one who likes to help people." She gave me a stern look, and I felt my face flush. I wanted to thank her for the lesson, but that would be a setup for another rebuke.

"You're right, Shar," I said, and sat in my discomfort.

Shar's words returned in those early days of grief and need. No one should ever, ever expect a widow to repay.

Let it go, Tally. Close the accounting book.

The twins hung the multicolored lights, ornaments, and silver garland and did a fantastic job. Several other close friends wrapped and delivered gifts that, per my request, cost under five dollars or were regifted. The tree blanket wasn't bare; I had eight gifts to open on Christmas morning, one per hour to draw out the surprises.

After writing and printing our holiday letter that year, I signed with a ballpoint pen, "Tally, and in memory of Jack." Did recipients see the dried spattering of tears here and there on the pages? I heard Jack's voice and laughter in my head. I felt his touch and occasionally smelled his cologne.

God, I miss you.

Immediately after Jack's passing, I lived the Alcoholics Anonymous motto, "One day at a time," although it was more like "five minutes at a time." I survived that first Christmas by counting the days until the holiday was over, when I could pack up the ornaments and lights. I yearned for a breather, a smidgen of calm, a time to heal.

On December 26th, among the half-priced holiday items in the local drugstore aisle, I watched clerks erect displays of cards, candies, and flowers for Valentine's Day. I glared at the workers and the merchandise. My fingernails dug into my palm.

Damn it, don't I get one week of reprieve, a whole damn day would be grand, from reminders that I am uncoupled?

Did we really need fifty days of hearts and red roses in every store, ads of smiling couples on exotic islands in the mailbox, and television ads of cooing couples buying diamond-encrusted jewelry? I wanted to hide until St. Patrick's Day.

In that first grieving year, I was alone at two weddings and two funerals. At the weddings, I missed how Jack and I always whispered along with the vows: "I, Jack, take you, Tally…" At the reception with tables set for an even number of guests, I sat next to an empty chair. At one funeral, I sputtered through one of Jack's favorite hymns while I heard his off-key voice in my head; neither one of us could sing well. He had a goal of taking singing lessons just so he could sing me a love song. As if in prayer, I bowed my head.

One of the memorials was for a former colleague of ours, a man who had spoken at Jack's Celebration of Life only six months before. When the minister called for those gathered to share memories of Roy, no one stood. I owed Roy and his family my words. I remembered fondly how Roy rambled his way through his speech at Jack's celebration, just as he used to carry on in staff meetings.

I felt air leave the room as I stood up from my chair and walked to the front. *What is she doing?* I imagined them thinking. But after years of addressing staff, students, and parents, standing at the podium in front of all these people was not a challenge. I took deep breaths and stood on steady legs. I grasped the wood sides of the podium and, avoiding the eyes of the room, said a short prayer.

Help me say the words, Bubba.

"Roy was a dedicated teacher. Computers were just coming into the schools, and he volunteered to teach the first computer elective class. I once asked him how it was going. He laughed and said, 'When I get confused, I ask one of the kids for help.'"

The crowd chuckled.

"He was a good man to teach our middle school boys. I heard him stop a boy from bragging with this simple advice: 'If you're that good, your friends will do the talking for you.' I had his daughter, Dannie, in class, and I know what a caring father he was to her.

You will be missed by many, Roy."

When I told Kate about that moment, she called it "showing up, with a large helping of strength and courage."

Lou Ann said, "My shrink would have patted you on the back for that. That was gutsy."

My inner accountant called it settling a debt.

Every Friday for over twenty years, I met up with three fellow educators, Joyce, Sandy, and Denise, in a coffee shop. We gave ourselves thirty minutes of conversation before we scattered to our different schools. I retired first, and still made the hour-plus round-trip drive to be there. I needed the "Friday Four." I loved these friends, and they knew and loved Jack, too. Three weeks before the first anniversary of Jack's passing, I brought big news to the morning meeting.

When I opened the glass café door, the aroma of cinnamon and burnt chocolate embraced me like an old friend. The room was already filled with people: the mother with a precious to-go cup in one hand and a child in the other, the student nursing a warm drink in a white ceramic cup while bent over his laptop, a hum of laughter and conversations rising like steam from various tables. I walked to the end of a short line to order my drink and checked the room for the others. I'd arrived first.

Over the hiss of an espresso machine, the young barista asked, "What can I get you today? The usual?"

"Yep, tea. Here's my mug," I said.

The café had an assortment of loose teas, and the baristas loved putting together different combinations for my custom drink. Whiffs of lavender and jasmine rose from my mug one week; chai and orange the next; or mint and something I couldn't identify, the combinations never tasted the same two weeks in a row.

I claimed a table, and one by one, my friends came in, ordered, and sat. Our spontaneous chatter and lively conversations had faded in the weeks since Jack's passing. I saw each of them glance at my face for some sign of how to proceed.

Denise asked gently, "How's Tally doing this week?" Her eyes held softness.

I blurted out, "I signed a contract yesterday to sell our house."

Cups stopped midair. I saw my friends exchange flashes of worry before diverting their eyes downward. I stared down, too. After a pause, they pelted their concerns at me.

"Are you sure?" asked Sandy.

"It's only been a year, Tally," Joyce added.

"And where would you go if the house sold?" Sandy's eyebrows furrowed.

I took a breath. Would I ever be one hundred percent sure?

The house was too big without Jack. The silence bristled; the memories cried out from the walls. "You think that a year or two from now it will be easier to let it go? I don't. But the timing is right, logically, and financially sound. That I am sure of. And in terms of where I'll go, I've got the cabin until I have a plan."

The cabin was two-plus hours away on the other side of the state, a drive over a sometimes impassable, snow-bound pass in the winter. But it was only June. I had time to work out those details. My friends gave me looks that said they had their doubts, but they didn't push me any harder to explain the decision.

The next week's announcement at the Friday gathering was even harder. Through tears, I told my friends, "I put Annie B to rest on Wednesday." I desperately wanted the dog's company on the first anniversary of Jack's death, but three weeks before that anniversary, it was time. The vet came to the house, put *our* dog to rest, and took her remains for cremation.

"Oh, Tally, what could be next?" Joyce asked, not really wanting an answer. "This is too much, Denise," a dog lover knew this loss.

"You poor thing, when will the big changes stop?" Sandy hoped for peace and calm for me.

I'm still not sure when they will stop, or if they ever will.

Months before putting Annie B to rest, while driving to a vet appointment in the quiet car, a day when I needed soothing silence rather than screeching music or talk radio, I questioned whether I could endure life without Jack. I watched the occupants of the car next to me at a stoplight: a couple in an animated conversation, hands waving in the air, mouths wide with laughter. As I pulled into a parking spot near the vet, another twosome walked hand in hand, heads leaning toward each other in tender conversation. How could I fill this huge crater in my day-to-day existence? All the leftovers, the "us" and "we" and "ours," where could I put them?

Waiting in the parking lot until the appointment, Annie B detested the smells of the vet office, so there was no going in early. I tilted the rearview mirror down. I saw reddened, tired eyes with dark rings underneath, a mouth that drooped at the corners, and cheekbones that had become more prominent with weight loss. I wanted the old me back. I wanted my old life with Jack. The more I saw that wasn't possible, the more I fought to make it happen.

The old me was a funny, spontaneous, creative woman. She was locked inside a dimly lit, small room, with a door that the new me pushed against, time and time again, begging to bring her out, to exchange places. After a few months of trying, the new me found the door unlocked, entered, and discovered the room was empty. The old Tally was never in there. She left with Jack.

My friends thought I was one tough cookie. They admired what I did and didn't do: I did attend our weekly morning coffees; I did show up to theater performances, soccer practices, and games. I didn't seclude myself in the house or run off to some rented room in an obscure spot in the world. I showed no new signs of self-harm, no scars on my arms from cutting myself. From the outside, I was okay. But a simple dust bunny broke me.

One morning, I stepped away from the dining room table, with all its bills, miscellaneous forms needing signatures, others to be read and reread for understanding, or simply tossed into the recycle bin, and, on the pretext of addressing my dust allergies, I pulled out the vacuum and headed up to our bedroom, cleaning carpet edges, the window frame above the bed with its dead moths and flies, and spider webs in ceiling corners. Jack usually held up the mattress while I vacuumed underneath, but I awkwardly skewed the mattress on the bed frame to expose one triangle of floor at a time. On the floor under the head of the bed on my side, the left, I found a dusty grocery store receipt and an old bookmark from the Cannon Beach bookstore.

How many of these did we bring home over the years, Jack?

I wondered what treasure I would find on Jack's side, and my heart began to race as I pushed the mattress to expose the floor beneath his pillow. With a deep breath, I stared up at the trees outside the window, then down to the floor. I saw a torn piece of yellow paper with a phone number in Jack's scrawl, layered with gray dust. As I reached for it, I saw something else pressed against the cherry-wood leg of the bed frame: a love card from me to him. It must have slipped off his nightstand and down through the slats. I pulled it out and read the inscription: "I will always love you." I wished I had dated it and pressed it into my chest.

Oh, Jackson, I miss you so much.

Wiping my eyes on the sleeve of my T-shirt, I placed the card on his nightstand.

Moving to clean beneath the foot of the bed, I leaned down to examine a thick bit of lint. Pinching a pile of dust and lifting it into the morning light, I saw strands of Jack's hair and Annie B's fur. A piece of each of them was alive in my hand, right here in the quiet of the room.

I pulled out individual hairs and touched Jack's reddish-blonde strands, and the silver ones that came later. There was Annie's fur, black on top with white at the roots. Holding strands to the light, like thin threads of glass, they glimmered. I was mesmerized. I had witnessed Jack's body being removed from this house, but this hair remained. The funeral-home technicians didn't take all of him. I twirled the hairs back and forth between my fingers, and a revelation came: I wasn't living in what I called "Pretend Land," a term I coined in therapy for the place where facts can be denied and one can imagine anything one wants. This life wasn't a dream. I had proof that Jack was here. And now he was gone.

Suddenly, my body folded onto the floor. How I longed for Jack and Annie B, the bodies from which those hairs fell. A damn dust bunny took me down.

"Pay attention," Kate's Post-it note said.

To dust bunnies? I thought, weeping.

"You vacuumed under the bed?" Lou asked. "Ya gotta be kidding me. I have piles of saved plastic bags, a Costco-sized box of toilet paper in the living room that's been waiting forever for me to put it away, and God knows what food has gone bad in the refrigerator. Vacuum under the bed? I'd have to find the vacuum first."

"Obviously, we had two different standards of clean," I teased her.

The truth was, I tried to keep the house in the same state as the day of Jack's death, in case he came home. And if he didn't, well, dust and dirt were two things I could control. So much of widowhood I could not.

Season after season, I pretended that life got easier, that I could handle widowhood, that I was living on. Life was happening for other people; friends and strangers were doing ordinary tasks, everyday routines, as if their lives would go on forever. I knew otherwise.

In my weekly recycling bin, wine bottles clattered together and rang like church bells, announcing my ongoing self-pity party. Typically, one glass was plenty and resulted in a light buzz. But on those dark nights, alone on the couch, shouting from the depths of my lungs, "Oh, God, I miss you, Jack," I sought cover and armed myself with a second glass. I felt poked, dragged, smacked, like a pro wrestler on television, the underdog, lifted off the mat, limbs flailing to hold onto anything but air, then slammed down by my opponent, spitting into my face, *This is your sucky life.*

A gulp from the glass sent a warm red wave down to my gut. My hand slapped the couch arm. I detested living for one. I took another swallow, jabbed my finger at the ceiling, and hissed, "Why me, God?" Took another sip. I abhorred the emptiness of the bed. I hated the quiet mornings. On and on the list grew as the glass emptied. Then it was time to head to the kitchen for a refill. My feet staggered across the carpeted room, hand grasping the dining room chair and bracing against the wall until my hips finally leaned against the dark green granite countertop in the kitchen.

"I hate my life," I slurred as I tilted the last drops from the bottle into my glass.

I miss you too much, Bud.

"You're a cheap date," Jack used to chuckle on our evenings out. "Don't have to buy you a lot of booze." A glass of red wine with dinner. Maybe an Irish coffee afterward.

"Cheap, but not easy," I would retort with a wink. I didn't like the sensation of being out of control: jumbled words, unsteady steps, whirling thoughts. The worst was the hangover, wasting the whole next day. An educator's weekend was always packed with errands, home projects, and schoolwork. There was no time to waste on nursing a headache and nausea.

Where was that rational, steady-footed woman now? Inside a wine bottle, hiding, numbing the raw edges. Even drunk, sorrow soured my gut, screams crowded my throat, and the yearning for his touch never softened.

Oh, Bud, this life is so hard without you.

I wasn't always kind to others in "The Afterwards." I wrapped my anger into icy snowballs and pitched them at the innocent. Once, arriving late to a social gathering, I hurled my fury at the hostess, who was a dear friend.

"How are you doing, Tally?" she asked kindly, meeting me at the door.

I unloaded. "Traffic sucked. Finding parking near this house sucks, I hate being late for a party, and, generally, this is par for the course, as my life sucks."

The stunned look on my friend's face stopped me. I didn't have the courage to backtrack and apologize in that moment, so I shoved my hands deep into my pockets and clutched a dark thought.

I hate myself.

When I became a school counselor years ago, a mentor advised me that good counselors could never commit suicide. How hypocritical it would be, given all the students I advised out of such a deadly decision, warning against "a long-term solution to a short-term problem." I was a model for those kids, showing how adults handled tragedies and heartaches. Suicide was not an option for me.

Grieving Jack's death, I nearly became that hypocrite. Many a time, I thought of killing myself, a quick and easy means to end this horrendous stabbing pain. Death was a means to silence the internal wailing and screams. I needed to stop the ghostlike memories of songs we liked, books we read, meals, and memorabilia that haunted me. *Burn them all. Quickly.*

But I was a good counselor, respected by colleagues and students alike. I wasn't a quitter; I couldn't let that be my legacy. Somewhere in my mind, I believed I could live through this hell. Jack would expect this of me, as I would of him if I had died first. Even in absentia, I needed his approval.

In a session with Kate one day, deep in what I called "my black hole," I recalled her Post-It note: *TELL YOUR TRUTH WITHOUT BLAME OR JUDGMENT.* I told her about my suicidal thoughts.

"Have you thought of antidepressants?" she inquired.

After thirty years of working with adolescents in the schools, I could rattle off the list of meds for ADHD, anxiety disorders, and depression. When conferencing with parents about medicating their kids, I always presented two sides of the coin. "Thank God for pharmacology," I'd say. "But ask your doctor and research the side effects and the withdrawal process before you decide."

Leaving Kate's office with a stack of antidepressant brochures, I read, compared, and decided. The side effects of headaches, loss of appetite, insomnia, and constipation, among others, scared me. Instead, I opted for a light box, more vitamins and herbal supplements in my daily routine, cut back on caffeinated teas and alcohol, get regular exercise, put myself outside in the sunshine whenever possible, continue journaling, and check in regularly with supportive friends. If I saw no results in three months, I would reconsider a prescription.

Days started with good intentions, but the sun set on unfinished tasks. I still wrote emails at two in the morning, mixed up dates, rushed late to appointments, and cried seemingly for no reason. As three months expanded into six months and inched into a year, I saw a pinpoint of light, something to crawl toward.

BE OPEN TO THE OUTCOME, the fourth line of Kate's Post-It note said.

For my third Thanksgiving without Jack, my brother Mark begged me to join him for Thanksgiving in Mexico, in the small coastal town of San Carlos, where he had a *casita*. I dropped off my new dog, an elderly Jack Russell rescue named "Anna," at the dog sitter's home. How easy for the dog when I called her, "Annie!" But she was an entirely new dog, with a new life. I, too, was ready for something new.

My Seattle flight stopped in Phoenix, where I caught my flight to Hermosillo, Mexico. There, I rented a car to drive to San Carlos. With no Spanish other than food orders at my local Mexican restaurant and numbers *uno* to *diez*, I clutched the steering wheel of the small compact hard, eyes flicking nervously to the mirrors to check for faster cars and commercial trucks coming up from behind, and glanced to the shoulder for javelinas and feral dogs. It was a four-hour drive on an unfamiliar highway with erratic traffic rules; as Mark explained, "Get out of whatever lane you're in if someone is riding your back bumper; use the shoulder if you have to." The trip was already an adventure and a challenge.

Mark and Lisa were still in Phoenix, driving down a day after my arrival; I had one whole day to fend for myself in San Carlos. First on my list was to hit a local exchange for pesos. I don't know if I got a good deal, but it didn't matter; I needed the money, and I was certainly a *gringa* in a new land. Next was a grocery store for peanut butter, bread, bananas, cereal, and milk. I dumped my new money on the counter before the cashier and let her take whatever was needed, thanking her for the coins she handed me in return. With supplies in hand, I followed Mark's incomplete directions. The left turns my brother had described should have been rights. I couldn't find the white fence or billboard he'd named as landmarks, and I traveled down the wrong unpaved, potholed lanes, passing the wrong pink and white adobe homes with dark red tiled roofs. With a good amount of swearing, I arrived, by luck, on the last street I tried, at his *casita*. I walked down the rutted dirt road to the neighboring home of an older American couple, who handed me a house key and a few frozen homemade meals from their freezer. I was set.

Mark was an Al Pacino look-alike, four years older than me and a head taller, with the tan of a longtime Arizonan. No one could doubt we were siblings: the same dark brown eyes and hair, straight noses, and thin lips. He still had a full head of hair, with gray strands penciled in.

I ran my hand through his hair. "Ooh, some grays in there, you old fart."

"You would have grays, too, if you didn't cheat," he retorted and swiped a hand at my head.

"Yeah, but I don't, and you do."

A warmth filled my chest to be with family. I missed spending time with someone who knew my history.

Thanksgiving was a day of misfit moments that accentuated where I was and wasn't. We ate soft beef tacos, not turkey and cranberries, at a nearby taco stand with a large open barbecue. The air was filled with the smoke of grilled beef. I wore a tank top and shorts, as did Mark and Lisa; in contrast, the locals wore sweaters and jackets, proving we were not acclimated to our surroundings. The only green in our meal came from the jalapeños, and I knew better than to try more than one. We sat outside, perched on plastic patio chairs and a wobbly metal table on a cement patio. Without city lights, Orion, the Big and Little Dippers, and other constellations felt close enough to touch in the warm Mexican air.

For four days, I walked or jogged the beaches, collected small, smooth, colorful rocks, read a book I bought at the airport, and ran errands with Mark. On my last day, I swam with dolphins at a nearby aquatic park. The weather felt healing, and so did my brother's company, how I missed the family tales we shared. I wished I could carry this sunshine back to the gray days of the Northwest winter. I wished Mark lived closer so I could get regular refills.

Mark and Lisa left to return to Phoenix, and I drove myself back to Hermosillo. I got lost finding the airport, and my heart pounded in panic as the minutes ticked closer to my boarding time. I recognized no landmarks and saw no signs with the international symbol of an airplane. I stopped at a convenience store, but my "¿Inglés?" only got me a shrug of the shoulders as the two male clerks murmured something between themselves. Could they see my frustration and panic, or hear me scream, "SHIT!" at the steering wheel once I'd climbed back inside the car? When I looked up through the windshield, a plane was descending overhead. I found the airport on time only because I followed its downward flight.

Thank you, Jackson.

I stood alone at the luggage turnstile in Seattle, surrounded by the hugs and chatter of people reuniting. My eyes moistened, my throat filled with envy, and my luggage felt heavier than before.

I miss you, Bud. You would have been here.

I found the shuttle to my parked car, picked up Anna from the dog sitter, and entered the cold house.

Our lunch plates were nearly empty. Water glasses had been refilled several times. The conversation still bounced around widowhood.

"For the longest time in the beginning, I wanted my old life back, the way I was with Jack. But I've changed. That woman doesn't exist anymore," I said.

After one final mouthful of rice noodles, Lou Ann swallowed, nodded, and agreed, "Me, too. But we're better people now. We get, truly get, grief."

"I wished I could have learned it all another way, and not through Jack's death."

"Nah," Lou Ann smiled, "We would have just kept poopin' along, doing what we always did. Unchallenged. Loss does that to you, you know, challenges you to your core. That's when you find what you're made of."

"We are survivors, aren't we?" I tipped my water glass to her in a toast.

"Yeah, something like that," she grinned and tapped her glass to mine.

"To whatever the future holds for us."

Raising her glass a second time, Lou Ann added, "As long as he's single, healthy, and not wanting a 'nurse with a purse.'"

I lifted my glass higher. "For all we've done in these last four years, we're more than survivors. We're thrivers."

"Yeah, something like that."

Chapter 20
Sex and Widowhood: Missing It All

My two fellow widows and I strolled into an urban café for a pre-theater lunch. Immediately after entering through the oversized metal and glass door, we heard soft jazz and the hum of conversation floating in the air around us. Amidst the rich cherry paneling and large windows that faced a busy Seattle avenue, a business-suited clientele was seated at tables already filled with plates and glassware. An eager server dressed in black pants and a long-sleeve black dress shirt with a contrasting white apron greeted us with a warm, "Welcome, ladies." Our heels clicked on the dark slated floor, telegraphing our arrival as we walked behind him to a vacant table.

We had met at a weekly support group for the widowed, where teary snippets of our stories were disclosed and bonds created. All three of us were in our fifties when we lost our husbands. Holly became a widow five years ago, and Lou Ann and I were only two years out. Our husbands had all died in their sixties, two after a long illness and one from a sudden heart attack. We were the survivors.

I wondered if Holly and Lou Ann had also struggled to find something adequate to wear to the theatre for the viewing of the musical" *First Date.*" The irony in the name of this musical hadn't gone unnoticed; to my knowledge, neither of us was seeing anyone. Without my husband, I didn't have a reason to regularly dress up, attend shows, or dine at fine restaurants. I'd lost my easy date. Did Lou Ann and Holly dig out dressy clothes they'd shoved into the back of their closets, long ignored in favor of jeans, sweatpants, and t-shirts? My indecisiveness was scattered on my closet floor: a blouse marked with a line of dust from more hanging than wearing, skirts that slid off my hips after so much weight loss following Jack's passing. Ultimately, I ironed my Sunday best slacks, cinched the belt to the last hole, and declared, *Good enough.* The last decision was footwear. I'd been living in running shoes and work boots. Although the two-inch heels added a dressier look, I knew I'd miss my flats if we didn't find a close parking place.

As widows, we knew there was a pile of post-death desk work waiting for us back home on our tables or desks, something new arrived every day, or so it seemed. It could all wait one more day while we took this time to enjoy each other's company. Who wanted to rush back to a quiet home?

In the center of our table sat a hummus and pita platter to be split three ways, and each of us had ordered a different salad so we could taste from each other's plates: arugula with feta, tortellini with fresh mozzarella, and spinach with roasted almond slivers. I smiled at the variety of tantalizing flavors before me, in contrast to the quick microwavable dishes I had been living on, overjoyed to be fed without dealing with shopping, preparing, or cleaning up afterward.

"You know the topic they never talk about at the meetings?" Holly peeked up from her salad to see if she had our attention, then diverted her eyes, poking at a cherry tomato on her plate.

In our meetings, tough discussion topics are common: handling adult children's grief, the reconstruction of holiday rituals, or the heart-wrenching removal of the deceased's clothing and possessions from the home. Of course, we discuss the stages of grief and practice naming our feelings: how to deal with anger and sadness, how to find sources of simple joy. But there was one thing we didn't talk about.

After hearing Holly's question, I restrained myself from appearing like a TV game show contestant, jumping from my chair and shouting the winning answer for our team, but I knew what she meant. Lou Ann's face lit up, she had the answer, too. The word loomed over Holly's head like a comic strip cloud.

Lou Ann and I blurted out together, "Sex!"

In her emcee role, Holly smirked and, with her fork and its speared tomato pointed at us, punctuated, "How. Right. You. Are."

Indeed, we sidestepped that topic in the support meetings, avoiding embarrassment and arched eyebrows, the shocked, *"Tsk! At my age?"* that might come from older group members. I felt such a twinge of envy when those members, in their seventies and eighties, spoke of their golden anniversaries. Jack and I reached only our silver. Who was I to judge?

During meetings, sex has been sidestepped with innuendos: "I still sleep on my side of the bed," or "I miss holding hands," instead of *I miss having sex.* Once, a woman's comment vibrated with such sexual energy that it silenced the room: "I wear his cologne to smell him on me." Many women confessed to the same, wearing their partner's shirt for that sensory connection. Men spoke of laying their wives' clothes under the covers, or on the pillow on their side of the bed. All of us had stepped into closets, hugged their clothes, inhaled the memories of our loved ones, and cried.

Someone might ask, "How do you handle the loneliness?" But that was the closest we got to discussing intimacy. No one said, *I miss getting laid.* No one wanted to admit that they might still crave an orgasm, the whole-body shiver from deep inside. Pheromones floated in and out between the chairs and across the tables in the room, calling us back to our bodies to remember the heat rising from our groins, the excitement of hands gliding down to pull hips to hips, and the smell of day-old sex. I haven't forgotten. I enjoyed lovemaking with Jack and missed the good sex we had before cancer and treatment ruined it. Perhaps some of my peers had negative sexual experiences and were relieved that, with death, they no longer had to fake enjoyment or lie still until a spouse was done. For them, death was a release from an obligation. But no one said such things aloud, the good or the bad, not in that room.

When the ratio is eight women to one man in our age group, a woman who mentions the need for sex looks as though she is waving a green flag at the eligible widowers, bellowing, "*Yoohoo! Over here! Pick me!*"

I was envious of the advantages of being a heterosexual male. Widowers can pick from a variety of sizes and ages, be choosy, be coy, while straight women are like the wallflowers sitting on the chairs at the high school dances, waiting for someone to notice them. Back in those days, we were trying to breathe in our constricting strapless bras, look cool, and hope our dresses stayed up over our total lack of breast development. Now, breasts were less of a problem than the liver spots, wrinkles, and need for glasses to see what was right in front of us.

In either case, I was clear where I stood: I still wanted it, the Big IT, which included the Big O. I am, and have always been, a physical being who enjoys her body in motion, whether racing the wind on my bike, playing on a soccer field, digging into the earth to plant a garden, or lovemaking. This is just who I am.

Until cancer came into our marriage, Jack and I touched each other often: running a finger across the shoulders when passing by, a hand on the arm when watching TV side by side, a stop on the staircase for a "two-step kiss," with me on the upper step. We held hands when walking together and made love on a regular basis. Treatment took his libido, and even when there was interest, what remained of his stamina was a "quickie" at best. We were both frustrated.

With his death, every time I rolled onto my left side, I was startled by the flattened sheets and undented pillow staring back at me. *There lies the memory of my partner and my sex life*, on that right side of the bed. The decline of my own libido, not wanting anything more than consoling hugs from friends, no one ever spoke about that in meetings, and I didn't start the conversation either.

After months of uncontrollable tears and deep grief, I began to pull the black veil off my body. If the support groups, held in the meeting halls of local churches, evaded any conversation with the word "sex" in it, imagine broaching the topic of satisfying one's own needs on one's own side of the bed. Nary a word. But privately, I wanted the pleasure my body could give. I had stored memories to reenact, making love with my absent husband, feeling Jack inside me. I kept our sex life alive.

As much as it was pleasurable to use my vibrator this way, typically tears followed. Opening my eyes after an orgasm, I saw the ceiling, not Jack. As if dunked into a cold bath, the post-orgasmic glow was extinguished as I remembered that sex was on the long list of things I now had to do alone. If I ever dated again, I realized, I could not have one man in my bed and yet another in my head. I had to put Jack out of the bedroom when being sexual.

I began to wonder what it would be like to have a new lover. After years of lovemaking with one person, starting over—the laborious, exploratory stage of telling someone where to find those erogenous zones—seemed overwhelming. Letting someone discover me: the right breast more than the left, the soft tickle of pubic hair, and, if all went well, the crying out ringing in the left ear of my lover. I know some men my age have…well…a functioning problem: what goes up doesn't stay there as long. Will we waste precious minutes on *not there, here, more, more, and what are you doing?* I imagine myself blurting out in post-coitus chitchat, "At your age, you still don't know what and where a clitoris is?"

Having sex with a new partner will entail knowing that lover's other lovers. I shudder at the thought of sitting in an examination room with my feet up in stirrups, being probed for the sample, and being told later, with the doctor's arched eyebrows and an air of condescension, "Ms. Reynolds, you have herpes," adding a little click of the tongue and a long sigh, "and you're how old?" Even thinking about this scene brings shame to my face, as if I were fourteen, radiating from my ovaries.

I'm too old for the bar scene. I'm not a part of a church, community group, or workplace. Thus, meeting like-aged men will be difficult. When I asked my little sister if she knew someone my age, she replied, "Sure, I know a lot of single guys. They're just too damaged to introduce them to you." That leaves online dating sites for seniors, a whole bag of trouble in my eyes: obscene phone calls, crude emails, and stalkers. But I know of Boomers who married someone they met on such sites. This could be done safely, being cautious with personal information, and meeting in very, very public places. Someday.

When I do date, I imagine young lovers at nearby tables will chuckle at us as we hold each other's veiny, bumpy, jointed hands, ogle into dreamy eyes behind thick glasses, and lean over the table to lay a quick kiss on wrinkly lips. Our snickering eavesdroppers will wonder what we could possibly be talking about on a date at our age. Best places for a senior discount? Stories about our grandkids? Maybe we'll get risqué and show a surgical scar or two. Maybe romantic meals will reflect the recent blood work-up: *"Gotta cut back on my sugars,"* or *"Cholesterol is on the rise. Fish for me."* The young folks will look at us and wonder, *"Does he buy, or do they split the cost of the Viagra?"*

When my silk slips off, it will be skin on skin, his on mine, his in mine. The quilts will be tossed aside; shared body heat will radiate between the sheets. A single taper candle will scent the room with vanilla and provide light enough to hold the moment together.

Back at the crowded restaurant, our desserts are on the table. Grabbing a bite of her cheesecake, Holly eyes it and shakes a forkful at us. "Why can't we have better snacks at our meetings, like this luscious morsel? Costco cookies and more Costco cookies every week."

I snicker. "When we can talk about sex at meetings, only then will the snacks become richer and sweeter."

Chapter 21
Shifts: Third Year and Still Forgetful

I felt lost in this new house for two years. It was like living in a giant jigsaw puzzle where the box showed one picture, but the pieces created something else. I tried to force the familiar into the unfamiliar and watched while the two fought for primacy.

The house was furnished with items Jack had never seen. There was the navy blue four-piece sectional, the fifty-inch television, too big given how little I watched, but it fit the wall space, the cherry wood bed, the dining room table, and the rainbow colors of Fiesta plateware that smiled at me when I opened the cabinet door. I moved through these rooms daily, yet everything felt too brand-new, as if still bundled in the manufacturer's plastic wrap. I wanted a home, not just a house.

I bought the kitchen dining table a few months after Jack died. It was my first major purchase without him, marking the beginning of my role as sole decision-maker; all items in the checkbook ledger would be in my handwriting from here on out. I saw the table while shopping with a neighbor. The thick circular glass top spanned five feet, perched on a base of four metal swirls. The four accompanying chairs had a question-mark metal pattern in the middle of their backs. The whole set called to me, something different from the oak table that sat eight, which *we* bought when we moved into the Bellevue home. The table was expensive, an extravagance, but I rationalized that I'd earned it, that I needed it. As if a table would soothe the pain.

What do you think, Jackson? I spoke to the air in the furniture shop as I ran my hand over the cool glass and blackened metal. *Should I do it?* In the silence, I knew Jack would have liked it, but only because I loved it.

And I did love it. Sometimes, in the dining nook of the new house, during the daytime hours, I felt like I was both sitting inside and outside. The nearby window's light shone through the glass tabletop onto the dark wood floor, onto dust curls, dog fur, and food crumbs, and, simultaneously, the outside trees threw their reflections next to my placemat. Here and there, inside and out. Almost magic.

One late spring morning, I sat at the kitchen table in my well-worn sweats, a second cup of Irish Breakfast tea cooling in my hand. The room was quiet. A red placemat, showing a week's worth of food stains, denoted my place at the table, but I did not feel present. My mind could not pull out a task from the long to-do list in front of me: a page filled with strikethroughs and additions, resembling a small child's crayon scribbles.

The early light in the back wetlands appeared like tossed bright green shards against the dark backdrop of limbs still in morning darkness. Robins, wrens, sparrows, and others gathered at the feeders. Grabbing seeds, they darted so quickly past the kitchen window that I saw only what appeared to be their shadows flying by before they retreated into the alders, maples, and cottonwood behind the house.

Anna was snuggled into her bed by my feet, settling into her "forever home," and her companionship softened the harsh stillness, much like Annie B's presence did after Jack died. Often, the difficult question is, *What do I do next?* It could be answered simply: walk the dog, hold the dog, play with the dog, feed the dog. The chandelier light cast a small shadow around her, an aura of contentment.

The chandelier was new too, brushed nickel with three snowy glass domes. It replaced the shiny brass chandelier I inherited when I moved in, whose bulbs lit the ceiling and left the table in shadows. This light was on a dimmer switch, as were all the lights that I touched in the morning. I have always detested bright lights, loud noises, and even conversation in the morning; I want everything to slowly unfold for me in those early hours. Of course, now that Jack wasn't coming downstairs to disrupt my quiet, years of insistence on morning solitude felt selfish; I had wasted precious time I could have spent with him.

Glancing at the dimmer switch, I recalled a shift with Jack in our first home, as he watched me put in a dimmer in my bathroom.

I'd been keenly focused on my project, in the zone, when I heard Jack shuffling back and forth behind me. "Need any help?" Jack peered over my shoulder as I stripped the wires in the outlet box. "White to white. Black to black," he advised.

"I've done a half-dozen of these. I know what I'm doing," I replied quickly, then added a polite, "Thanks for the reminder," hoping this would soothe his bruised ego.

Jack's new wife was doing what he thought of as his job, a "manly" task, and she didn't need his help. I was an independent woman, and Jack would soon see I was eager to learn more about remodeling.

"Teach me how to do plumbing," I begged him later. Eventually, there were lessons on framing, sheetrocking, running a backhoe, and roofing, until we were quite the team.

Last week, chatting with a widowed neighbor on my new block, I shared my current projects, painting, installing new garage loft storage racks, and other endeavors. My neighbor listened, then shook his head and told me I was "too self–sufficient," warning that I "might scare off most men."

Stunned at his frankness, I had no response but a thin smile. *I don't want that man in my life*, I thought. Any man who would be intimidated by my home and yard maintenance skills wasn't for me. Why should I ask for help from a man when YouTube, Google, and helpful employees at the hardware store hold almost all the answers? When I couldn't find help, I solved the puzzle myself, sometimes by trial-and-error-and-error-and-error, but eventually, the task was done. I needed to believe that I could do this, especially now that I was a widow. I heard Jack's encouragement in the saws and drills. *You can do it. Go slow.*

Yeah, Bubba, you taught me well.

Are you disappointed that I sold our house, Jackson? After all that work we did to make it ours? But surely Jack understood, I couldn't stay there without him. Those walls held his sweat, swearing, and sweet soul; I would forever feel his ghost there. I had to, Bubba, I had to get out.

Placing my palms on the glass of the table, eyes closed, I tried to pull Jack from our old home onto the chair next to me. In this smaller kitchen, his nearly six-foot, two-hundred-pound frame appears in a forest-green bathrobe, almost wedged into the space between the counter and oven range. I hear the rattling sounds of beans grinding, smell the brewing coffee, and smile in response to the gurgle from the pot. Jack stands over a bowl of batter, then moves to the stove to flip pancakes. Unlike our early married mornings, today these pancakes are neither too thick nor burnt; he's had plenty of practice. Maple syrup, margarine, and peanut butter are set out on the table. Now Jack is in the chair next to me, holding my hand for grace before the first bite. As we eat, I hear newspaper pages crinkle.

I opened my eyes, an empty table. I take in the evidence of my cold cereal breakfast this morning. Who does pancakes for one, anyway? Leaning back into the chair, the hard metal poked my spine, and I heaved out a sigh. The room felt smaller, as if that fantasy had sucked in the walls and clouded the windows. I realized that time was altering my memory of Jack; when I closed my eyes, I saw his grey-and-blond moustache through an out-of-focus lens, smile wrinkles smoothed out around his eyes, those robust Scottish shoulders and broad chest. When I imagined him, I conjured a healthy young Jack, not the thin, chemo-bald man at the end of his life. I was grateful for this.

With payday yesterday, the top of the list was what I called "The 3 Bs:"

- Balance checkbooks

- Budget

- Bills

Jack was such a procrastinator, and I'd often resented his lackadaisical attitude when it came to this monthly chore. I had no tolerance for anything that could ding my credit rating.

"Screw yours up," I would say, "but if I get dinged..." I let the sentence drift off in an unspoken threat.

Jack came into my life with a much lower credit rating than mine, which caused the bank to initially balk at our first home loan application. My rating saved us. He accused his previous wife of not paying their bills with the money he gave her, a story I bought until it was bill time in our household.

"What's the VISA bill doing among the wrestling mail?" I asked, waving it in the air like a fan.

Jack was deeply involved in the local wrestling officials' organization and had piles of mail from them on numerous spots on his desk, mixed in with miscellaneous letters, team schedules, bills, and meeting times. I kept orderly files in a cabinet. I had a mail slot for "bills" and "correspondence" in the kitchen, and kept folders for income tax deductions and important documents in my study. Frustrated by his piles, I finally bought a new bin and labeled it, "Jack's."

Then I saw that the bill was due in two days. "Are you going to pay it soon?" I stood at the entry to the basement TV room, at a safe distance, though I wanted to be a foot from his face.

"I know when it's due. I'll get to it later." He returned to the game on TV.

I stepped into the room. "How much later?" I kept myself from adding color. *How much* fuckin' *later?* That would only escalate an already heated situation.

"Later." With his eyes forward, the words passed through hardened lips.

"It's due on Wednesday." *Fuckin' Wednesday.* Tension sparked between us.

"I know. I said I would get to it *later*." His jaw tightened, and those neck tendons popped up and then down into his shoulders. I left it be.

The envelope with the check to VISA waited for a stamp until Thursday morning.

"What the hell, Jack? It was due yesterday."

"They give a grace week or two, you know."

We repeated this same fight for different bills, again and again. There were fights about where to file bills. Fights about writing checks and mailing bills on time. Fights about unknown charges on the VISA, which never seemed to get paid off, regardless of how much of our modest teachers' salaries went towards it. I nicknamed him "Quick Draw" for how quickly he pulled that charge card out to get a tool, new drill bits, a new wrestling officiating bag, and flowers delivered at my school. I rarely declined his offer of a meal out, even though I knew the charge would irritate me in four weeks when the bill showed up with a balance still due.

Our shared checkbook ledger held more than numbers. Now it was all mine. I didn't miss the fights, yet fighting would mean he was still alive, here, digging in his heels with me.

A robin sat on the deck railing, startled when I rose from the table to toss the last of the cold tea into the sink. *Sorry, you red-breasted beauty, come back.* I'd brought Jack's laptop to the kitchen table so that the birds could keep me company with this morning's task. I needed to boot up the laptop and open access to my bank account.

My index finger did not immediately register a cursor in some spots on the pad, and I thought of Jack's impatience with technology. He used to poke and scrape and curse at the computer, thinking that if he pushed harder on the pad, the machine would execute what he wanted faster. Hearing the swearing from his study, I knew the computer was taking the brunt of his ignorance.

Here I was at Jack's computer, his fingers once danced over these same letters that I touched. I wished for his warmth to rise from the keys that touched my fingertips. To be touched and touched back. But these keys were cool. And filthy.

Jack wasn't a big cleaner. Dust, floor dirt, smelly bed linens, well-used towels, and his piles everywhere; he just didn't see housekeeping as something needing his attention. Only I saw it. When I got overwhelmed on a Saturday morning and yelled, "This place is a MESS," he was willing but clueless. "What needs to be done?" "What do you want me to do first?" Eventually, I would organize a master list and ask him to choose a task while asking myself if I could ignore his half-ass cleaning job, or if I'd be going behind his back to redo the job later.

Obviously, regular cleaning of the laptop keyboard wasn't on Jack's chore list. I got to work scrubbing the grimy keys before realizing I was further removing proof that he was once here. *Can't you keep it the way it was? A memorial to Jack, the slob.* I didn't like my compulsive side that fought leaving some things as he left them. I didn't like the computer keyboard cleaning spray that evaporated quickly and hurried me. I didn't like the feel of the cleaning cloth as it skipped over the keys. I didn't like the telegraph-like sound the keys made when pressed down. I didn't like the clean white alphabet that glared back up at me when I was done. But then, I didn't like my life right now either.

A neighbor back at the old house, a friend of both of us, told me to be careful when I opened the computer: he knew of a man who left his wife a final letter there. Would that be Jack's way of saying goodbye to me, a letter completed months ago when he was healthy enough to get up and walk the fourteen steps to his study? Maybe on a soccer night when I was gone for several hours. Maybe?

A part of me wanted to find those final words of love on a saved computer file, words that would rip open memories like wrapped Christmas presents. Waiting for the screen to come to life, I heard my pulse in my ears, quick and strong. My right hand hovered over the keypad, waiting to double-click a desktop file titled something like *To my wife, Tally.* What would he express? Would I finally get those words I craved back when he was dying? Maybe I could let go of the anger at the silence he gave me while he talked to other family members about how much he would miss them. This could be my private moment with Jack, even if the words had to be typed. *That's OK, Jackson. Anything, anything, to fill emptiness.*

But after twenty-six years together, I knew Jack well, and this wasn't his style. He bought store-bought romantic cards with lines of borrowed prose to profess his love and added, *I adore you,* and *forever my divine love,* in his left-handed chicken scratch. I took a deep breath and checked the screen in front of me. The desktop was blank.

Move on, Talle. You knew a letter wasn't there.

I sighed and navigated to my online banking account password.

"What is your wedding date, mm/dd/yyyy?"

This online security question should have been easy to answer. After all, I chose it from the options, thinking the date would be forever etched into my mind. But today, three years after Jack's passing, I stared at the blinking cursor ticking off the seconds, panic escalating with each flash. What was the year? "October tenth" was easy to remember because of its rhythmic" *Ten-Ten,* " but the year.

What was the year, damn it? You should know this!

Leaving the kitchen table, I rushed down the hall into my study to the wood file cabinet I brought from the old house. The bottom drawer rattled on its rails as I pulled it open, and I yanked out the file marked "*Vital Documents*." This familiar folder contained all the documents various institutions requested for closing and transferring items into my name: his death certificate and community property agreement, my name change, and our wedding license.

For months after his death, I'd kept the folder in its clear waterproof document case in the back of the car since I never knew when or which form would be needed at which corporate or government office. That file was like a vampire in the backseat, unseen in the rearview mirror but present, sending chills down my spine. I detested every page of that file, and I relished the day when I took it out of the car and filed it in this bottom drawer, in the far back, out of sight.

But I must have filed the wedding license in another spot; it wasn't here. I didn't remember doing that, but I didn't remember a lot from those early months. So much paperwork. So many tasks. So little brain, given the fog that began when I rose in the morning, swirled around my every step and every thought, and surrounded me until I retired in the evening. Back then, I created file folders marked with big black letters and placed them around the dining room table:

"Death Certificates"

"Life Insurance"

"Celebration of Life"

"Accounts/Titles to Change"

"Social Security"

"Tribe Business" (Jack was part Blackfeet Native American, on his mother's side)

"Wills/Community Property"

"Obituary"

"Funeral Home"

"State Ferry System," with its process for burial in the Puget Sound

"Bills"

"To Do," with its calendar for checking off tasks

Out of the chaos, I'd attempted to order. If I walked to the table and immediately filed whatever was in my hand, it was there later. But I found random items dropped in the kitchen, bedroom, and office, or a letter from the state pension department that had sneaked into the "Calls to Make" file.

Still standing in front of the file cabinet, I thought of another form that might have the wedding date in it: Jack's community property agreement. But, damn, all personal information was redacted, per legal protocol. I knew that; mine was the same way. Where else? Damn it. Think! Sitting down in my desk chair, I pressed my hands on the sides of my head. *Think!* As if I could squeeze out a solution through the holes in my spongy head.

I wished I had the year engraved into my wedding ring, as I did in his, fearful that he would be the stereotypical husband who forgot anniversaries and other important dates. Jack was never that; he always made reservations and gave me flowers and a card with printed words of love and commitment. Always. He didn't need to check the ring to remember the date. Now I was the one who needed the reminder, but Jack's ring was stored in a safe deposit box in town.

I pieced together what I did know: I was twenty-eight when we married; we would have celebrated our 27th anniversary if he had lived a little longer; and it had been three years since his death. My feet tapped the floor, and pen drummed on the desk as if that would beat basic math skills back into me. I made error after error until I finally reached *1981*.

I am so sorry, Jack. I never thought I would forget our wedding day.

Through tears, I navigated back to the table and computer, security answer in hand, only to find a message,

You have been disconnected from this banking transaction.

Too much time had elapsed.

Chapter 22
Storms: At the Cabin Alone in a Storm

Five miles up the canyon, the hot breeze rippled the dried grass of the hills, and deer and elk nestled in the ravines away from the Eastern Washington sun. The quails and rabbits hid beneath the wild roses and low-growing trees. For years, Jack and I watched the wildlife move across these four acres as it changed colors, from the bright greens of spring to dry summer tans to winter white.

The property felt different with Jack gone, as if someone had shaved off the tops of the hills and shushed the males of the coveys. As if the wind had stolen the scent of the wild roses. Emptier were the cabin rooms. And I wasn't the same woman either.

But still, at the cabin, the quiet still soothed and renewed. On clear nights, the Milky Way arched directly overhead, and my favorite constellation, Orion, stood alert in the sky. I missed Jack at sunset, as the small pricks of light dotted the darkening blue. We used to sit on our Adirondack chairs on the wide front porch we built, an open bottle of red wine between us, Annie B on her pad at our feet. We played our evening game of counting the awakening stars until we counted twenty-one.

"There's the first one," Jack pointed to the southern sky. Playing the game for years, we knew where to focus our eyes for the early stars.

"Number two is at nine o'clock from that one," I chimed in, "and three is above the hill."

One by one, we went until twenty-one stars were spotted. So serene. So simple.

Until one night, alone after his death, a storm scarred the land and my peace.

Softly at first, the thunder caromed up the canyon like the rumble of a large diesel truck. Far away, lightning sliced into the dark gray sky. More and more rumbling came, until it sounded like a caravan rolling up the street, vibrating against the cabin. The light flashed hard into the windows. I counted, "One elephant, two elephant, three elephant," boom! The storm was less than fifteen miles away. Faster and brighter, and louder. Another flash followed quickly. "One elephant, two elephant," boom! Ten miles. Before I could count after the next flash, the thunder immediately replied. Overhead.

Little Anna quaked in my grasp as each vibration rattled the framed art on the walls and the glassware in the cabinet. Nature's timpani clashed with the sounds of Yo-Yo Ma's *Bach* on the stereo, my futile attempt at hiding the storm from my poor dog. Did she hear my heart race against hers while I held her to my chest to soothe her? With her wide brown bug-eyes, she begged as if I had the power to stop this.

I usually loved a good storm, but this show was different, louder, stronger, and closer than any other storm. Worry whirled inside my chest that the cabin would be like Dorothy's house, plucked up in the storm, eventually landing in Oz.

Each lightning strike struck at my ignorance and lack of physical strength. If something happened to the cabin tonight, could I handle it? I envisioned myself climbing a ladder to do a makeshift repair with a tarp, rope, and duct tape in the hard rain, feeling my way around with a small flashlight held in my mouth, getting soaked to the skin.

I was terrified that I could lose everything we built.

The storm would have been an adventure with Jack. Popcorn popped, divided into two bowls, and two only because Jack's large handfuls emptied a bowl before I had my share, and on the guest bed where the television and DVD player were. With old Annie B packed against one of us, as she didn't like thunder either, we'd watch movies until the lights went out.

Eventually, Anna and I heard the thunder slip away to another town. We went outside, and I advised her to make it quick, the clouds were threatening. The rain began just as we stepped back in. Small taps on the wood deck, the windows, and the metal roof. Drops became faster, bigger, and harder. Suddenly, torrents of water hit the front of the cabin like a fire hose turned on the house. Unlike the flash floods of my Arizona youth, this rain did not stop in an hour. It rained long after I turned off Yo-Yo Ma's baroque tunes. Long after we went to bed.

I slept through what the locals called a mud flood. Water raced down the sides of the ravine and gathered against old clay walls. Before morning light, one more drop was too much, and the dam collapsed. Yards and yards of mud and stones rushed down the ravine, sloughing off walls and floors in its wake, and collected more force and strength.

Early morning, I woke to the sounds of big earth-moving equipment, male voices shouting instructions, and the beeping of commercial vehicles backing up. Dressing quickly in shorts and a sweatshirt, I slipped on flip-flops and ran outside. And prayed to the cloudless sky.

Please, nothing wrong, Bubba, I've got people coming today, the people who bought a stay at the cabin at the auction.

I gasped.

I stood before a completely blocked graveled driveway. The red clay mud was piled a foot high in places. Some tree branches and entire root systems tangled in the roadside barbed-wire fence; others passed through the fencing onto my property. Metal fence posts were nearly bent in half. The mudslide continued across the driveway, through the lower acre, where a swath of debris appeared like a muddy highway twenty feet wide, forty yards long. It slid under the single-wire property fence before stopping somewhere on the lower adjacent land. Dozens of the fifty-pound retaining wall blocks had traveled as far as fifty yards; corners poked up to mark their final resting spots in my driveway and in the lower acre. Rocks of all sizes were everywhere, large ones like icebergs, unmovable when I tried to kick them loose. Where grass once grew, several wild rose bushes appeared as if planted upside-down, like large chicken feet pushed up from the mud. Tossed here and there were long tree branches.

The two tall poles on either side of the driveway entrance—one with a black metal sign that read "Reynolds" and a quail family silhouetted above—survived unharmed, though in the mud they had shrunk from six and a half feet to only four feet tall. I forced a chuckle and recalled a disagreement on a hot morning regarding those poles.

"Nice job, Jack. You were right in using the larger bags of cement on those poles. More work then, but you were right."

I wiped my tears on the sweatshirt sleeve. This mess was huge. Overwhelming. Too big for one person.

Flip-flops were the wrong footwear. With each step, the mud suctioned my shoe off. I balanced on one foot several times to pull out the stuck shoe and put it back on without stepping barefoot into the mud. I was in no mood for yoga stretches or red-stained feet from the clay. Backtracking, I returned to the house, put on a pair of knee-high cement boots, and resumed my paralyzed stance in the driveway.

All I could do was look.

I saw Kermit across the road, whose landscape blocks dotted my land, and Rich from below, out near their homes. We all had the same stymied look, hair skewed from bed. They each held a morning coffee mug with rising steam. Both knew Jack and knew I was widowed.

"Are you OK? Do you need anything?"

Trying to be lighthearted and feigning confidence, I replied, "A Valium? Shot of scotch, maybe." They laughed; I grinned and shrugged. What could I ask for? I whispered to the ground: "What I need is my husband back."

While the county crew cleared the road and Kermit's entire driveway, I raced back in, fed and walked Anna, grabbed a piece of toast, tossed the sweatshirt for the t-shirt, and headed back out. With its clay base, the mud would be difficult to move when dried. The sun crested the eastern hills, and sweat gathered on my back and around the rim of the "Life is Good" baseball cap. I needed a piece of him with me and wore his hat. But more than ever, I needed his hands and his wisdom. His absence pounded at me like last night's thunder.

I had a couple arriving in five hours who had won a two-night stay at the cabin in an auction to benefit support groups for the widowed. Unfinished chores included beds to make, towels to put out, a final dust and vacuum, packing up myself and the dog, and leaving the guests to their privacy. But now there was a thirty-foot driveway to make accessible.

I made slow, too slow, progress with the tractor bucket and a square-point shovel. The reddish clay mud was thick and heavy. I stopped frequently to move limbs or push large boulders to the side. I stacked Kermit's fifty-pound retaining wall blocks, the ones I didn't have to dig out, for him to retrieve later in a drier part of the property. The buckets of mud I dumped were small, as I wasn't skilled using the tractor for anything other than mowing, stacking cuttings onto the burn pile, or dumping small rocks around the perimeter for fire protection.

I needed help and saw only one solution: the county men in the street. I sloshed through the mud of the driveway, climbed over the entry mound, and walked toward a big husky man in a well-worn, once-white t-shirt sitting in a large county dozer clearing mud. I waved at him. He shifted the dozer into neutral so we could hear each other.

"I need some help," I said, pointing to my driveway. "Could you move that mound of mud at the entry and the first few feet of my driveway, please?" With my tractor bucket (and my skills), I would need dozens of sweeps and buckets to move the mud, while he could do it in just three.

"Yes, Ma'am. Let me finish here," said the man. As I walked back home, I imagined him thinking, *The little woman is way over her head in this disaster.* Did I look pitiful on the blue tractor, out of place for a woman in this small rural town? *Man's work,* I saw in his eyes. *Where's her man?* He probably stepped across some regulation forbidding county machinery on private property to help this little old lady. Lord knows I felt small and old.

He moved the mud with two bucket sweeps.

Years before, I learned how another local man thought of this "little woman." Jack and I were in the local hardware store, a man's bastion if there ever was one, whose proprietor knew every item on the shelves and how to repair or replace just about anything. Jack had done the ten-minute drive into town several times over the years for a few bolts, a box of deck screws, electrical connections, and other miscellaneous small items.

"Can I help you?" the fifty-something man asked as he walked down the aisle toward the gardening section where we stood. He wore silver-framed glasses that matched his thinning grey hair, and his girth held many post-work beers on a body no taller than my five-foot-five. I noticed that his eyes were on Jack, as if I weren't there.

I stepped forward so I stood in front of Jack. "I need a water timer for the garden. Do you have any?" The garden was my project, my love, and I wanted the timer.

He turned directly to Jack and said, "They're over here."

I was stunned. *What just happened?*

"I asked the question," I bellowed at Jack in the car back up to the cabin, "but he gave his answer to you. Did you see that?"

Jack remained quiet.

"Did you see that?" I asked again.

"Didn't notice," Jack muttered to me.

He probably thought it didn't matter much whether the answer was given to him or to me. And maybe it didn't, until now.

"Come on over later," Kermit yelled at me from his driveway, "and look in my garage. You're not gonna believe it."

Two hours later, I rinsed the mud off the tractor and shovel, picked up Anna from inside the house, and carried her the fifty yards from my front door to his porch. Closest to the ravine, Kermit's property took the brunt of the slide. The mud plowed its way through the back walls of his two-story, four-car, metal-sided garage, dammed against the front wall, then busted out. Mud filled the bed of his pick-up truck. I knew by the handlebars, side mirrors, and headlight poking up through the silt where his motorcycle was parked. I sighed with sympathy for what a mess he had on his hands. Leaving that garage, I thought, *Thank you, Jackson. It could have been worse.*

Jack got credit for making my life easier. My personal angel, that's how I thought of him, who watched out for me. *Help me here, Jack,* when I was late and I needed green traffic lights on a long city street. *Please, please, make Boomer start,* as I turned the tractor key for the first mow after a long winter rest; the grass was high from a wet spring. Right now, I just wanted him here.

My midday guests arrived at a cleared street, an open entrance, and a good-enough driveway. I tossed them the key to the cabin and left. The lower-acre clean-up was for another day.

I survived the storm, not a disaster I could either anticipate or prevent. The mud flood wasn't because I forgot to turn off a switch, replace smoke detector batteries, or check tire pressure. But standing in the cabin before leaving, a childhood memory surfaced: I saw my mother. With her hands on her hips and her body like a snake ready to strike, she growled at her four young children, all under the age of thirteen.

"Well, someone did this mess. Who did it?"

Every mess had a guilty party, whose responsibility was to admit fault quickly and clean up. In my mother's house, innocent older children often took the blame to stop the yelling and save the smaller ones from the first slap.

Not my fault. I did nothing wrong.

That small little girl's heart thundered in my chest, anticipating the sting of a palm across my cheekbone.

Not my fault. I did nothing wrong.

Not mine, but Mother Nature's.

I spent hundreds of dollars to shore up the cabin, trying to stay ahead of the next storm. A plumber set the new water heater in a drain tub; if it leaked, water would be piped down into the crawlspace and out to the front yard. The unused dishwasher, with its dried-out rubber gaskets, was removed. Individual turn-off valves for the hot and cold water were installed for each bathroom and kitchen sink, fixing the cheap, shortcut plumbing done by the modular home manufacturer.

How close was I to another flood? How long could I keep the pieces together before the dam of maintenance and repairs broke into my savings?

"One elephant, two elephant, boom!"

"*Stay in the here and now,*" Jack chided me while I lay awake one night. "*All will be okay for several more years.*"

I shooed him off with, "Easy for you to say."

If the mud flood was the worst thing that was going to happen, I knew I could stay, but I was given no guarantee. Before the mudslide burst out of the ravine, the dam held gallons of water, little rocks, shrubs, and tree leaves. Small stuff, joined by other small stuff, and more small stuff, until the walls gave way. So it was with my life.

Mistake after mistake, oversight after oversight. Small stuff needed my attention and pulled me from one end of the yard to another, both at the cabin and at the house.

The tin roof of the entryway's little birdhouse had blown off.

Jack's truck needed new shocks, and my Baja needed new spark plug wires.

Anna needed a dental cleaning.

The pictures from my last trip were still in the camera.

While I was in the kitchen one night, the back patio motion-detected light went on. Startled, I saw a rat toying with the bird feeder. Rats in the backyard.

I left an expensive pair of bifocal sunglasses somewhere. I busted a clock beyond repair when I forced a new motor into its frame. I ordered the wrong size water filters for the cabin. The wrong headlight bulb for my car. I forgot to winterize the scooter at the main house, and without an additive in the gas tank, the remaining gas clogged the carburetor. I left the interior car light on at an airport parking lot and returned to a dead battery.

The small stuff was surely adding up to my own personal mudslide. In the silence and stillness, I waited for the next storm.

Chapter 23
Two: The World is Built for Two

Rage pulsed from my clenched jaw out to my fisted hands. I wanted to stomp, throw, and kick to the far corners of the garage all the unpacked contents of a newly purchased Costco compost bin. *A compost bin, for God's sake!* Such an odd object to arouse my wrath. The four black plastic panels became easy targets for my punts. The bags of nuts, bolts, washers, plugs, screws, and other miscellaneous hardware, which I'd separated by size and purpose and lined up compulsively in neat columns like tiny toy soldiers, evenly spaced apart so I could pick up one at a time, waited to be snatched up by my furious hands, flung at the walls, caught in a toddler's tantrum.

Just days ago, I stood at the Costco compost display and imagined happy worms and rich mulch breaking down the clay soil in my garden beds where the rhododendrons, cherry trees, and bulbs were struggling. In my head, the plants begged, *Buy it! Buy it!* Once I got the bin home, dressed for this warm late spring morning in a holey T-shirt, well-worn black shorts, and old running shoes, I knelt on a gardening knee pad on the cement floor. I was excited to assemble this contraption, which my ecologically minded and garden-loving self had always wanted. My sweet old miniature rat terrier rescue, Anna, rested on a dog bed a few feet away. We occasionally glanced at each other.

Pieces organized and in place, space made on the floor for the three-by-three-foot finished product, I turned page one of the manual and read:

"Two adults required for assembly."

Two. But I was alone.

I wrapped my arms around my ribs, struck by sorrow mixed with red anger. I rocked a familiar sorrowful chant: *I miss you so much, Jack.*

Nearly three years since his passing, I missed Jack with every step of this project: from Costco to unloading the box in the garage, to the assembly. If Jack were here, I'd read the instructions and he, glancing over my shoulder to see the pictures in the manual, would attempt to throw pieces together until his patience dissolved into profanity.

"Slow down, Bud. Let me read. Geesh," I'd bark at him.

With a long huff, he'd assert, "They never write these manuals so any fool can do it."

The compost bin broke me, but other situations caused me to falter. Food, buying, preparing, and eating, shifted my thoughts from the present into the past. What *didn't* go into my shopping cart was as painful a reminder as what did: a package of tortillas, a six-pack of a local microbrew beer, barbecue sauce, and salsas. I replayed our shopping rituals and conversations and found myself oblivious to fellow shoppers muttering, "Excuse me," as carts veered around me.

I once stood frozen in the middle of the aisle with a can of clam chowder in my hand, but it wasn't my hand that I saw. It was Jack's. He held two cans, comparing back and forth their labels for which one had the lowest fat and sodium contents to satisfy his wife's health-conscious demands.

I think this one is the best, he'd say.

Show me, I'd respond.

Shopping for one was taxing. With a shopping list, I sauntered down aisles and cringed at cans and bags plastered with the detested phrase "Single serving." My produce bags held fewer apples, carrots, and bananas, the days of Costco-sized food purchases were long gone. At five-foot-five, I couldn't reach items on the top shelf; I missed his almost six-foot height. Closing my eyes, I saw him smirking down at me through his mustache as he reached up and heard his tease, "Shortie."

The items I loved that he only tolerated, Brussels sprouts, turnips, the makings of stuffed green peppers, and my breakfast cereals felt heavier and landed louder in the cart. I tried to enjoy the food I prepared, but his absence dulled my taste buds.

After three years, my denial was no longer surrounded by a cement wall; I had chipped away at it each week in my therapist's office, and now it was thin, almost translucent, after many months of living alone. Time was a healer. I found myself smiling more often, occasionally roaring with laughter provided by little Anna's silly antics; those moments cleared my dusty lungs. Who belly laughs alone? I no longer expected Jack to join my laughter from the other room, but he was still the first person I wanted to talk to about just about everything. I still spoke to the walls, the ceiling, and the sky.

I accepted that he wasn't coming home. But I avoided our favorite espresso stands, as well as a pho café, breakfast spots, and Red Robin, for years. Until one day, a hot mocha sounded too good. From her window, the familiar barista greeted me. Esther was a twenty-something gorgeous brunette, a single mom, who used to show us pictures of her toddler whenever we asked.

Her manicured eyebrows arched when I drove up, and she sparkled, "Where have you been?"

Where would I begin, I thought. "Oh, just super busy and cutting back on the sweet stuff."

Esther stooped down in the window and peered into the empty passenger seat. "And where's your husband?"

The answer stuck in my throat. This was not the place or time to speak of Jack when all I wanted was something warm and comforting. She waited for my answer. On a long exhale, I said to the steering wheel, "He died."

I wanted to shift gears and leave before my drink arrived.

Esther dragged out each word, "I… am… so… sorry," and turned away.

"Me, too," I said softly, and held back tears.

Moments later, she handed the steaming, warm cup out the window. I grabbed it and placed it in one of the two cup holders between the seats. I extended a five-dollar bill and my punch card to Esther. She waved off my cash. "This one's on me," she said with reddened eyes. "Take care of yourself, now."

The drink soured before the first sip.

A few days after the compost bin purchase at Costco, a song of ours ended on the radio, and I whispered to the windshield, "I loved you so much."

Stunned. *"Loved?"* The tense rattled me. When did I push Jack into the past? When did this "new normal" quietly slip into my brain and let him slide further away? What else was I losing?

"Will you need help in loading this into your vehicle?" the clerk asked at the checkout. This three-foot-by-four-foot compost box would fit in the back of the truck, but I didn't have Jack's strength, who could easily lift the box in a bear hug.

I tossed a white flag into the air. "Yes," I said to the male clerk with beefy arms, "I need help loading it. Thank you." *I'll need help unloading at the house, too,* I thought. I heard the reality dipped with self-pity in the words.

At the loading area, the cart with the compost bin was parked at the edge of the truck gate. Store liability prevented the clerk from helping with any part of tying the box down in the truck bed. The responsibility was all mine. How much easier and quicker this task was with two, when one of us was on each side of the truck, tossing the rope from one side to the other, rather than what became a cumbersome rodeo event. My tugs, pulls, and knots in odd places worked, but contrasted with the fluidness and simplicity of the task when Jack was here.

I learned to get heavy items out of the truck, new book cabinets, new toilet, by slicing open the boxes inside the truck bed and laying out the individual pieces on the open tailgate. Back and forth from the truck, in and out the front door, and up and down stairs, I carried one piece at a time.

Plenty of people offered, "Call me if you need help, any time." But often, help was penciled onto friends' calendars with an invisible asterisk: *If nothing else comes up.* I begrudgingly learned to be patient, praying to the heavens, with fingers crossed, that my need for help coincided with someone's schedule on the same day. I often waited until someone got home from work in the late afternoon before I could complete a simple five-minute project that I started in the morning, because that last step needed multiple sets of hands. When help did finally arrive, I stockpiled two-person chores: "While you're here, could you hold that cabinet so I can screw it into the wall?" "Would you hold this shelf so I can mark the wall for mollies, please?"

When the washing machine failed on a Saturday, two months after Jack died, I made nine calls for help. Worried about how much money had flown out of the checking account, I had opted for a used machine.

Monday evening, call #1: "I saw your ad for a used washer on Craigslist. Is it still available? Super, I desperately need it… No, I don't have anyone to help load it… Yes, you gotta take care of your back. Will you give me a couple of days to track down some help?... Thanks."

Monday evening, call #2: "Katy, is your husband around this week to help get a washer for me? Mine died…. Oh, that's OK, I understand. I'll try a neighbor up here."

Monday evening, call #3: "Hey, Bill, my washer died. Will you be around any time this week to pick up the one I found on Craigslist?... Oh, where on the coast will you be staying this week?... Love that area… No problem. Have a wonderful time."

The phone got too heavy to dial another number. *I so miss you, Jackson,* I sobbed into the receiver.

Tuesday morning, call #4: "John, are you and Jamie working this weekend?... Yeah, I need a favor. Can you two help me on Sunday, say around noon, to pick up a washer I bought on Craigslist?... Sure, no problem, get back to me after you call him, please. Thanks. Tell Janet I say 'Hi.'"

Wednesday afternoon, call #5:

"John, any word yet from Jamie?... Oh, good. I'll bring the address and the check on Sunday to your house. I'm meeting Pat there to go to a show in Seattle... We won't be back at your house until late afternoon. Is that OK?... Here's my plan: I bring Jack's truck up to your house, you use that to get the washer, and bring it back to your house. I'll drive it home after the show on Sunday. The washer is only about 10 minutes from your house, and I'll have the directions for you. Any questions?... Good. Again, thanks so much."

Wednesday afternoon.

"This is Tally, who wanted your washer. I just got confirmation that my friends can pick it up. Do you still have it?... Great. So, Sunday around noon works for you?... Sure, check with your wife. When's a good time to call you back?"

Thursday morning.

"One o'clock is better than noon? Sure, let's go for it... Yes, my friends will have my check... No, I won't be there, as I have another commitment that afternoon..."

Thursday morning. I left a voice message.

"John, the guy selling the washer wants you and Jamie to pick it up at one, not noon. Does that still work for you two?... Give me a buzz when you get Jamie's OK, will ya?"

Thursday evening.

"Pat, we have a slight change of plans for Sunday's show... Yes, yes, you're still going, but my washing machine died... I know, bummer. I found one on Craigslist. Denise's John and Josh will pick it up for me on Sunday. I will drive Jack's truck up, they will get the washer while we are at the show, and then I can drive the loaded truck home later... You have no idea... Can we use your car to go to Seattle?... Yes, we'll still meet at Denise's. You're a jewel. I owe you a drink afterwards."

Friday afternoon.

"Hey, Great Neighbor Guys, before you drive off, I have a favor to ask. My washer died, and I need the old one moved out of the basement, help with unloading the one arriving on Sunday back down there, and then put the busted one back into the truck so I can take it to a recycle place. Can someone come over Sunday late afternoon, or even early evening?... Cool... What's your favorite beer?"

Nine phone calls, one across-the-cul-de-sac conversation, and seven days for a washing machine replacement. I missed simple and easy, quick, and now.

Later that summer, with the compost bin in place (after I snagged a neighbor after work for two minutes of his time), I built a sixteen-foot-long trellis for a purple-blossomed clematis to run along the fence line. Any piece of wood shorter than three feet I could handle easily, but the longer pieces required pre-drilled holes where a second set of hands would have held the board for the lag bolts or nails. The two upper long boards were two-by-six sixteen-footers and entailed braces, clamps, and grunts until I got them leveled and attached at the seven-foot mark on the three fence posts. Jack and I would have had it done in a day. Alone, I spent four days. But I did it.

Without Jack, it was no longer "*Two Adults Required*," but me figuring out how to live with the parts and pieces of the slowly disassembling "Us." Just me, with my living-on manual opened to a solitary page of instruction: "One adult required. Do whatever needs to be done. Ask for help. Get going."

Four years later, a neighbor drove his truck to a local hardware store to pick up a purchased 30" x 50" x 21" garden shed and brought it to my house. We lifted the box from the truck and placed it in my driveway. He drove off. I sliced open the cardboard and laid out the individual pieces. I carried one or two shed pieces to the backyard.

I opened the manual. First bold line: "Two Adults Needed."

Yeah, right, I chuckled to myself. *Can't do that to me twice.* I had it completed in a day. Alone.

Chapter 24
Falling: Skydiving for 60th Birthday Adventure

I will be sixty in a few days. Five years and a few weeks without Jack. A Leo who learned to walk her kingdom alone.

I once thought I couldn't live another hour without Jack. Not a week. Not a month. Every year, on the first day of January, I stood before the kitchen corkboard with a pushpin in hand to hang up a new "365 Days of Puppies" calendar, *our* favorite calendar. Every year, I tossed the old year into recycling, the remnants of a year without Jack.

The silence wasn't as loud as it once was, but the emptiness remained so. It pushed back and tripped me up at odd moments, so unexpectedly. Reading the obits one day, I said aloud, "Oh, Jackson, Ray died"..." My voice trailed off when I saw the room was empty, and a long, sad sigh escaped my lips. With a shake of my head, I whispered, "But you probably already knew this." I returned to the paper.

Five years haven't erased much. Jack still strolled beside me when I walked the dog. I asked him about decisions I had to make, or to help me process the ones I had made but later questioned. I winced then smiled when I saw his favorite items on grocery shelves, like pepperoncini and local micro-beers. I still raised my wine glass to the air and said our toast, "To the little ones and us and Annie B," before my first sip, although a different dog, Little Anna, snuggled on my lap.

I slept in the middle of the bed.

After Jack died, I continued our tradition of birthday adventures without him; this year, I went skydiving.

Even if Jack were alive, this would have been a solo adventure. Experiencing heights in this fashion was not to the liking of Jack's guts. On my two parasailing stunts in Mexico, over the bays of Puerto Vallarta and Mazatlán, Jack watched from the ground while I was strapped into a parachute and pulled behind a ski boat. Two years after his death, while I floated over Egypt's Valley of the Queens in a hot-air balloon, I knew he would not have enjoyed being by my side in that basket.

For a birthday adventure, I arranged for Jack to sit in the cockpit of a WWII fighter plane, alongside the pilot, for a thirty-minute flight. On the ground later, he admitted that his breakfast came up his throat on a couple of turns and loops. It was a thrill for him, but that was the only birthday adventure that prompted Jack to say, "Let's not do that again." No way would he have skydived.

I drove alone to the small community airport. As I got out of the car, I heard Jack in my head: "*Crazy, you're fuckin' crazy.*" I heard his chuckle and saw him shaking his head in disbelief.

My brother Mark said, "Anyone who jumps out of a good airplane is fuckin' nuts."

Maybe so. As a child, I loved jumping off the backyard swings to see how long I could stay airborne before landing. This adventure was my adult version of being airborne for more than two seconds. This was the thrill I wanted.

After signing the liability release forms, the first-timers were given instructions. We practiced the fall position on the floor: on our stomachs, arms up and bent at the elbows like we were being robbed, and legs spread with knees up at ninety degrees to the floor. In a few minutes, we would be doing this up there. I heard my pulse in my temples.

On this warm August morning, I opted for the jumpsuit, the official garb of jumpers, and a pair of their goggles, which solved my worry that my contact lenses might fly out of my eyes. The other jumpers included Jason, my tandem partner, who stayed in his cargo shorts and T-shirts. I may not do this again, so I went for 100% of everything and anything offered.

Jason was several inches taller than my five-foot-five frame, with a barrel chest that made him appear heavier than he was. He greeted me with a firm handshake and a toothy smile. A soft breeze sent waves through his full head of black hair. How much experience could this young guy have? He stood beside me while I pulled on the gray nylon jumpsuit, and we walked toward the plane.

"So, Jason, how did you start skydiving?" I really wanted to ask, "How long have you been doing this? And have you had many parachute mishaps?"

"Friends bought me a jump for a birthday gift. Been hooked ever since."

"And how long ago was that?" I asked. Smiling, he stared directly into my eyes and, addressing what he probably knew was the foremost concern of every first-timer, said, "I've done hundreds of jumps since then." I smiled back.

I was cinched into a harness that was similar to the one I used when getting on the roof: loops around my legs, loops for my arms, and a pair of two-inch straps across my chest. A man pulled on the straps until they were tight against my body and tucked in the loose ends. He double-checked each strap's tightness with a tug. I watched Jason put on his own harness and parachute. He walked over to me and slipped his fingers under my straps to check their tightness, with a casual, "Looks good." *Gawd, I* hoped *so.*

We waited in the warm sun until the plane arrived, and sweat gathered in my armpits and waistband. Maybe the jumpsuit was too much. Standing in line, I felt, from behind, again, tugs on my straps. Jason.

A shiver crept down my spine. Why so many tugs? If something went wrong, would these straps save me? *Swallow. Breathe. Trust these guys. Jason doesn't want to lose his customer or splat into the earth any more than you do.*

Once inside the plane, the pilot motioned, like a maître d', where I should sit on the aluminum floor of the plane, facing the back. Jason sat behind me, and I, between his legs, looked at his hairy knees, maroon socks, and well-worn hiking boots. No butt pads, no seat belts. Just the floor and hairy knees. I got a whiff of cleanly shaven-man scent when Jason first sat, that sweet yet earthy smell, but now it was overpowered by the interior's mixed odors of hot metal and a musk resembling a moldy canvas tent. There was probably a coating of nervous sweat from first-time jumpers on the silver metal interior, too.

One of the solo jumpers grabbed the cargo door handle and, with a big pull, the door slid along its track and slammed shut. Like a horror film, the click of the lock signified that we were trapped. Hostages. No one would hear our screams over the plane's engines. One of these people could be a mass murderer; they could throw us all out that door, without our parachutes. There was no escaping. My anxiety heightened.

Skydiving was *really* going to happen. I was fuckin' nuts.

The engine revved and, through the window on my left, I saw that we were moving toward the runway. The plane paused on the asphalt. The engine got louder, and I felt its vibrations in the soles of my day hikers and my rear end. In what felt like ten seconds, I watched the land disappear, replaced by nothing but blue as we moved toward our designated altitude: 13,500 feet.

I climbed many trees as a youth. As an adult, I braved heights many times, stapled and hammered down felt underlayment, cedar shakes, and asphalt shingles on roofs with Jack, crept toward the edges to clean out gutters, and brushed out the woodstove chimney pipe before winter fires. Caution was always there, whispering, "*Be safe*," and I focused on each step and motion. No daydreaming. I wasn't one to look down and panic.

Except one time.

"Look at the wall! Look at the wall!" Jack's plea rose in the brisk January air. He stood below on the driveway, and I stood frozen in place near the top of an eighteen-foot ladder. "One step at a time. Just move one foot down," he encouraged, although I heard no optimism in his voice. His words sounded clipped and laced with fear. Unable to come up, this loving husband had only his words with which to rescue me. I alone had to make the descent.

"I…can't…move," I stuttered to him as if even my lips were frozen.

I had gone up to the roof, stood on its flat section, and swept off the pool of water that had leaked into the house. I inched my way off the roof and back onto the ladder. I took two more left and right footsteps down, let go of the roof's edge, and grasped hard onto the sides of the cold aluminum ladder. With my hands and feet secured, I made a crucial mistake: I looked down.

"Listen to me," Jack called from the ground below. "Look at the wall. Don't look down."

"I…can't…move," I repeated.

My own voice sounded muffled in my ears, as if I were wearing a headset. My heartbeat pounded into my ribs. I closed my eyes. But it was fear that locked out thinking: I could not command my knees to bend and step down. I was terrified. My muscles and bones were locked still. Per Jack's instruction, I opened my eyes and stared at the brown wood channel siding through the silver rungs. I watched the worm-like beads of rain that reflected the gray sky race down the wall. One drip after another slipped out of my sight to the ground below.

When I tried to see Jack below, oh, *I knew better*, my vision collapsed into a long tunnel. At its end, through a small circle of light, was the driveway and Jack, no bigger than a small boy, calling up to me.

I stared back at the wall and clung to the cold metal ladder. I feared a blast of wind would pry loose my grip and throw me to the ground below. *Hold tight! Hold tighter!*

We both knew that it had to be this way, I on the ladder two stories up, and he on the ground with a foot on the first rung to keep the ladder feet planted firmly on the driveway, wet after the torrential rain. The eighteen-foot ladder had been adequate at our previous house, a fixer-upper with one floor plus a basement. But here at the two-story house we bought just two weeks ago, the ladder was three inches shy of the roof edge, even when stretched to its maximum height.

Our new house had three sections of roof: cedar shakes over the garage in the front and over the living room and kitchen in the back, with a strip of flat hot tar at the peak between. In this rainstorm, water had pooled on the flat section and wiggled its way into the house, dripped from the ceiling, and partially filled the clear glass globe of the ceiling light. The leak had to be stopped.

The trip up had been harrowing, too. With each step up to a new rung, my left foot following my right foot, the ladder arced toward the house under my weight and then returned to a straight line. When I got to the middle of the ladder where the two sections were locked together, the ladder shook and sent tremors through my body. *Right step, left step, wait for the ladder to stop quivering.* It felt like walking on a rope bridge, with its sways and pauses. Right step, left step, stand still until the ladder stops quivering.

An unwelcome mist began. Beads of water gathered on my hair and dripped down my neck. I gasped when the first chill rippled down my back and mixed with the sweat there. I inhaled the cool, clear air. The rungs of the gray ladder shimmered, silvery, with the mist. *Think about what you're doing.* I grasped tighter. *Don't slip.* I placed the arch of my foot solidly in the middle of each rung. *Focus.*

Step firmly, stop, wait.

My right hand reached up, grasped a rung, and pulled my body up, while my left hand held a construction-style broom with orange, hard bristles, the tool I needed to push the water off. The broom dangled like a pendulum and banged against the side of the ladder. With each step, it sent small shock waves into my hands and feet.

Step up, ladder bow, broom bang, wait for stillness.

Step up, ladder bow, broom bang, wait for stillness.

Only ten more feet to the roof edge.

I leaned into the ladder, and it pressed back into my chest, hips, and thighs. I expected bruises tomorrow.

Reach higher, grasp the next rung, pull up, and step up. Reach higher.

Please, God, don't let it rain again.

Near the top of the ladder, my head even with the edge of the roof, I shifted my right arm from a rung to hug the ladder from behind. I brought the broom out from the back of the ladder and inverted it so the bristles were eye level and the pole pointed downward. With a grunt, I pushed the broom over my head and onto the roof. I gave the pole an extra push to scoot it further, hoping for a clear path when I stepped on the roof.

Now I had two hands free, but four rungs remained until I maxed out the ladder's length. *Step, bow, quiver.* With three rungs left, I grabbed the edge of the roof and placed my right elbow on it for leverage. Two rungs left. Standing tiptoe on the last rung, I was high enough to bend at the waist, over the edge, and onto the roof. The first jolt: my chest and outstretched arms landed in a pool of frigid rainwater that soaked quickly through the front of my jacket and shirt. Shivers rattled to my core, and I gritted my teeth. I pulled my left knee up onto the roof, and my jeans soaked up more water. Another jolt. My right toe, the last connection to the ladder, pushed off, briefly suspended in the air while I crawled army-style on elbows and knees across the puddle and away from the edge.

I whispered into the water, "Thank you, God," and stood up.

I took several deep breaths. *Center yourself.* Surveying the view, I saw the top of the trees in the back greenbelt, evergreens, and leafless maples. I heard no birdsong in the trees. Ah, the winter silence. The cul-de-sac was quiet, too, with neighbors sheltered from the rain inside, a few front porch lights still on. The three mid-twenties male renters across the street, who were often outside working on their cars, must be inside with a football game. From there, I saw the edge of Lake Sammamish. A realtor might call this a "peek-a-boo lake view property." *But from the roof?* I chuckled to myself.

With broom in hand, I scanned the roof for structural damage. "I don't see where the water is running into the house," I called down over the edge.

"We'll have to tarp it for the winter," Jack called back up. A chore for later, after we've purchased a *longer* ladder.

"Look out below, here comes it," I yelled, and swept cascades of water into the air.

With the last swipe, I tossed the broom down to Jack, lay flat on the roof, and inched my way to the ladder for my descent.

"I'm still here," Jack called up to my frozen body on the ladder. "Now, listen to me. Listen to me." I knew that commanding voice, the one Jack used when he thought I was ignoring him. "I'll catch you if you fall. You're safe."

My two little sisters used to call me "Spock," after the character from *Star Trek,* whenever they heard me insist, "It's only logical..." during our arguments. The sheer illogic of Jack "catching" me sparked my synapses. Falling fifteen feet, weighing one hundred-thirty-some pounds, I imagined that Jack would break my fall and my fall would take his life, blood oozing from a head wound as my weight slammed his into the asphalt. His last sound would be a grunt as the air was knocked from his lungs, and I would hear the crackling of bones contorted into odd angles.

Hell and be damned if he's going to die saving me, I thought. Hell, if that was going to be my last memory of Jack, imploring him, "Hang on, Bud, help is coming," as I rushed into the house and called 9-1-1, all because I panicked on the ladder. I, who wasn't afraid of heights, until today.

My thawing brain told my heart that everything was under control. *You can do this*. I took a deep breath and then another. Warmth began in my toes and spread until I felt the hard rung under both feet: up through my calves, around my knees, and thighs. The ladder still sent chills into my hands, but I could twitch my fingertips and loosen my grasp.

Do it!

From below, I heard his cheers. "One foot. Good. Now another. Good, good. I'm still here. You're doing fine. Almost there, Talle."

Finally, both feet on the driveway, I fell into his waiting arms and sobbed out my terror. "You did it," Jack cooed into my ear. "You're safe. I'm here."

Around twelve thousand feet, Jason leaned forward and said into my ear, "I want to put the straps on that will tie us together. Are you ready?"

This was really two questions in one: Was I ready to be strapped to him? And was I ready to go through with this adventure?

With a thumb up: "Sure am."

Three sets of straps were crossed over my chest, and Jason yanked hard on them. We were bundled together. Tightly. Securely. *How can he even breathe with my back squished against his chest?* I felt Jason tug again on my straps, and on the new ones that banded us.

From the front of the plane, the pilot yelled that we were nearing thirteen thousand five hundred feet. Jason pointed to the two women standing by the cargo bay door, one with her hand on the handle, and said, "Those two are working towards five hundred solo jumps." The woman pulled the door open, and air rushed into the plane. Or did air rush in from a collective gasp of the rookies?

Oh shit! This is really, really happening.

"Why five hundred?" I asked, attempting to hide the drumming pulse in my chest with casual conversation, could he feel it? I wanted to project that *I was cool with that open cargo door and nothing but blue sky out there.*

"That's how many they need to do to become an instructor," he answered. I like that number, five hundred.

The six instructors must have conferred together before we left the ground and figured out the order of the jumps. Because Jason was the heaviest and now had my weight on him—which was why they asked for my weight on the registration form—we were assigned to go first of all the tandems. Jason explained that ordering the jumps by weight prevented any mid-air collisions with lighter, and thus slower-descending, pairs.

Whoa! How much faster will we go?

But I liked the idea of going first: not waiting, not watching other people, not witnessing any of their anxieties, and not having any preconceived idea of what an instructor does to exit the plane. Ignorance was good. Going first was fine with me. But I still wondered, how *much faster?*

Amidst the roar of the engine and the whoosh of air at the open door, I felt a tap on my shoulder and heard in my ear, "Are you ready?"

So many divers chicken out right at this point, Jason had told me earlier on the ground. It would be okay with him if I changed my mind. *Not me.* To get this close and not jump? *No way.*

"Yes," I said, with a strong nod to be sure he knew I was all in.

Years later, when I recalled the experience of jumping out of "a good plane," to quote my brother, my nerves would reenact this moment, going from butt firmly planted on the metal edge to dropping out the door, falling into nothingness, and watching the ground come toward me. My heart re-enacted the fall, regardless of where I was. This was the most alert and wide-eyed I had ever been, more than at any other time in my life, including my wedding to Jack (I knew it was the right move), parasailing (flying over water, what was the worst that could happen?), and crucial win-or-lose plays at championship softball or soccer games. This jump was recorded permanently in my body, in every single cell.

I wasn't really scared, just more anxious about the unknowns. No other experience compared, other than jumping off those swings as a kid, for reference. On a deeper level, I was keenly aware that I sat at the line between living and dying a horrific death. I pushed the limits, like the time I rode behind a friend on his motorcycle, speeding over a hundred miles per hour. That rush of speed, the air pounded against my helmet, legs, and arms in defiance of mortality: I knew if we crashed going that fast, by the time I stopped tumbling along the asphalt road, nothing would be left but a hundred-yard skid of blood, skin, and bones; only my head still intact inside the helmet. Yet I wanted to go faster. Something wild in me wanted to test and live at the edge.

Some might say I had a death wish, a wild desire to be with Jack. Not so. I wanted to live fully, fuller than ever, because I had learned how quickly life changed. In a second. How death awaits. *Live with no regrets* was my mantra. If I ended up sitting in a convalescent home in my ninth decade of life, I would admonish myself if I had missed opportunities. *I wish I had skydived when I was younger. I wish I had jumped.*

I wanted to live life now.

The two wanna-be-instructor women jumped first. Appearing as casual as if they had walked out the front door of their homes, they stepped out of the plane. And, swish, they were gone from sight.

Oh God, that was quick.

Jason and I, strapped together in a vise-like grip of straps, crab-walked to the open bay door. The air was surprisingly warm as we sat there with our feet dangling over the metal opening. Like a racing sprinter, a pulse ran through my body. I was at the edge.

Between this plane and the ground below was thirteen thousand five hundred feet of empty space: no clouds, no birds. Clear blue sky. Nothing but Jason and me, our straps… and a parachute that should open. At the exit door, I felt both the pull to lean forward and peek, and the panic that pushed me back into Jason, back into the plane.

I leaned.

Looking out, I saw where the horizon met the tops of the Northwest mountains. *Not so bad.* I wasn't dizzy or queasy. Slowly, I bent forward and peered down at the ground where we would land. I saw small patches of green and tan farming squares, highways like long gray snakes, dots of cars, and the squares and rectangles of rooftops.

You're right, Jackson, I am fuckin' crazy.

"Ready?" Jason yelled.

"Let's do it!" I yelled back. Jason pushed us out, and I fell into space.

Oh my God! This is incredible.

We soared like eagles, silently, for thirty seconds in our practiced position, the "free fall." Then Jason pulled the chute cord, which shot us straight up as if we had done a bungee jump. Head rush. The chute appeared like a huge ivory umbrella overhead. I expected to hear a whoosh of the air, but I heard nothing. Were we really falling that slowly? So quiet.

Jason did a "corkscrew," where we twirled around and around like we were attached to a maypole. We ended with a five-minute slow glide to the ever-nearing ground, where more details, people, billboard images, car colors, and small outbuildings became clearer.

Nearing the landing spot, I heard, "Knees up," and I brought my knees up to my chest. Jason's feet touched the grass first, and then his legs collapsed so that I landed softly on my rear.

He released our straps. I turned and squealed while I danced around him, "I did it! I did it!" His grin matched mine. I experienced everything possible in a tandem skydive. Such a head-and-heart rush, from the edge and back.

Back up in the plane, seconds before Jason pushed us out, I turned my focus to the heavens and felt close to Jack in this vast expanse of air, as if I could see his smile, those blue-grey eyes, and a full head of youthful red-blond hair again, just behind the blue canvas sky. A small prayer came to me. I asked Jack, my birthday adventure partner of twenty-six years, *Get me down safely, will ya, Bud?*

Chapter 25
Birdhouse: Our Cabin, My Refuge

Alone at the cabin for these five years without Jack, on the four acres of land we bought ten years ago and tamed, I pondered the question of friends. *Why do you keep the place?* The work to maintain land that grew tall with deep-rooted weeds, wild bushes, and trees that flourished on nothing but morning dew in the hot summer months and two feet of snow in the winter. The arthritis in my left thumb gnawed at me while I held a simple notepad to write a shopping list for the town, and my right hand showed the beginnings of carpal tunnel, those small needle pricks in the fingertips when I gripped the pen. As dominoes tumble down a line, I wondered in what order arthritis might attack the rest of my joints. Shoulders? Hips? Knees? Too much yard work yesterday for one person, my hands said. My back agreed. It was easier with two. How will I, a sixty-year-old widow, maintain the place when the pain becomes too much?

Up five miles of a hilly canyon with tall grass and sparse pine trees, I sat in the kitchen, warmed my hands around a clear glass mug of Earl Grey tea, I loved the color of tea, and watched the morning sky brighten as if on a slow-turning dimmer switch. The sun will peek over the eastern hills soon; the deer will run across the land and hide from the heat of the day under trees in hollows, but not before nibbling on the apples I threw along their worn paths. The birds began to call to each other.

At our weekly coffee gathering, Sandy asked why I go by myself. "Isn't it lonely?" I told her the land and its inhabitants were my company. I returned to listen to the cackles of blue-jacketed jays, the hawks' shrills while they glided overhead, the songs of the warblers and starlings as they darted between power lines and trees. I watched male quails lead their coveys as they scurried on the ground between the low-growing shrubs. They were the reason the place was nicknamed "The Birdhouse." I came to feel the breeze whoosh off the canyon walls as it cooled the midday sweat on my back. In the spring, the wild roses and the caramel scent of newly cut hay will sweeten the air. I deepened my roots in the soil.

But there's another answer to her question.

I am not alone here.

Out here, I closed my eyes and easily envisioned Jack. He is up on his royal-blue canopied tractor, nicknamed "Boomer," wearing that olive "Life Is Good" baseball hat with its sweat-stained brim, his work jeans with dried smears of paint and caulking from past remodeling projects, and his favorite faded navy flannel shirt. (I take that shirt off the hanger in the closet and wear it, too.) He grins and waves when he sees me, and I wave back.

"Are you thirsty?" I gesture, tilting back an invisible glass. Cold beer for him and iced tea for me wait in the refrigerator. He shakes his head and goes back to mowing until I hear the tractor engine die, see him hop off, and watch him walk to the deck. We sit with our legs over the edge and enjoy the view down the canyon.

Ralph, Jack's father, from Spokane, once visited us at the Birdhouse. While watching his son mow, he remarked, "It's in his blood. His grandfather and his great-grandfather were farmers." The Reynolds men and their tractors, I watched genetics at work.

I hear the tractor rumble out there. Occasionally, the mower blades clip a rock, and a "Damn it!" or other choice words travel up to the cabin. Ah, there he is.

Annie B is out there, too. She runs her property, follows the scents and fecal droppings of deer, rabbits, and neighbors' dogs and cats that cross property lines, or lies alert on her red pad on the deck. When her black fur becomes too warm, I might find her with a dangling pink tongue in the shadow of the bench or under the deck on its cool dirt. She stays out on guard duty until we all go in.

Meanwhile, I garden in old cotton shorts and a tank top and dig up the rocks that seemingly grow faster than the carrots, tomatoes, radishes, and other vegetables. Later, I walk ahead of the tractor, pick up exposed rocks, and throw them into a wheelbarrow or the tractor bucket to be dumped around the house for fire protection.

With the heat of the day, we come inside to the air conditioning and lunch, quick quesadillas, or peanut butter sandwiches. There he is in his rocking chair with a book or the sports section. Maybe a nap. In the cooler late afternoon, we return to finish whatever was started in the morning.

Hours later, freshly showered in clean clothes, we prepare a simple dinner together: pasta with marinara sauce, local barbecue plates, or simple cheese, fresh vegetables, and Italian bread. Always simple. Afterwards, one of us washes, the other dries, and we both put everything away.

We sit on a wooden bench assembled from a kit: several four-foot 2x4s inserted between two green plastic side frames. Our thighs touch when we sit together. Or we sit on the pair of Adirondacks and matching ottomans we purchased one summer; the chairs, always close enough that we can hold hands.

In the warm, clear evening air, with Annie B at our feet, we reminisce about our yesterdays. We retell, again and again, how things fell into place: the serendipity, how a local wrestling buddy of Jack's drove us up this canyon to find a parcel of land for sale; that the local Wenatchee dealer of modular homes had one left of last year's model and offered a lower price. The neighbor two houses down the canyon sold his older tractor for a fair price to us. We replaced it with Boomer years later and passed that older one to another neighbor up the canyon.

On the deck, we make plans for the tomorrows we think we have.

Inside, the wine bottle is corked and the glasses rinsed. Standing in the kitchen, sexy grins and raised eyebrows pass between us, that look that says, *I know what you are thinking. Do you want to…?* Rested from the fatigue of the workweek, rest that made lovemaking longer and more enjoyable, we begin with passionate kisses and hands reaching for sensual areas. Clothes are pulled overhead, unzipped, discarded, and we enter the bedroom fully aroused and ready. I see it all in my mind's eye.

I made the two-plus-hour trip to the Birdhouse because Jack was there. On one side of the driveway, in the corner of the "L"-shaped retaining wall, amidst the six rows of abode-colored blocks, a single gray block in the third row marked where a third of his ashes rest. Another third was released off a Seattle-to-Bremerton ferry in remembrance of our first date when we bypassed the "Do Not Enter" sign, went into the captain's tower, and watched the docking. The last third was buried in the sands of Cannon Beach, Oregon, our favorite summer getaway town. Two rows above him, behind another gray block in the wall, were the ashes of our dog, Annie B, his first puppy, our only dog together. They were here with me at the cabin.

Yes, I am lonely, but not alone.

Sounds traveled far in the canyon: the coyote called to its pack, local dogs answered, horses and cows snorted and whined, and, higher up the canyon, heavy dozers and backhoes worked on a new foundation or well. The echoes from either up or down the canyon sounded as if they came from the edges of the property. In the cool early evening hour, I heard neighbors still mowing and hammering, and I smelled barbecue meat carried on the wind. When outside, I often eavesdropped on their conversations and ached for those casual exchanges between couples, something about a chore, a silly dream, even the angry *What were you thinking?* And, reminded of a life I no longer have.

Although the neighbors frequently invited me to join them for dinner or drinks, I didn't. I was cordial and thankful for the rural hospitality. The across-the-street neighbor, Kermit, who was about my age, often made occasional off-colored jokes, I think, just to see me blush, but I rarely did. He drove his ATV over and regularly checked for break-ins when I was away. Gary, who lived two properties down the canyon, was an older silver-haired man with a younger wife. I think he sought excuses to get out of the house some days. He cleared the driveway entry during the winter so I could drive in. If I ever needed help, I could stand on my deck and shout. Someone would hear me and come.

Like a good neighbor, I gestured a hello and smiled at passing cars, kept the gully out front clear of garbage, and kept the wild grass and weeds mowed low to keep fire hazards at a minimum. I offered my neighbors tomatoes, rhubarb, sweet pumpkins, and other harvested items from the garden. Every Christmas, I took a holiday-wrapped box of truffles to the five homes that were within a quarter mile of me.

But I came to the Birdhouse for the quiet. I yearned for the dirt under my nails, a comfortable chair by the window, and a good book. I watched the sun dip behind the western hills while I sat on the deck bench. I missed the tickle of a hand as it glided up my arm and the slow kisses. The emptiness burned. A long sigh gathered, whirled inside my chest, and slipped out into the cooling air.

Will my death be like Jack's, one that slowly overtakes me, or an unforeseen tragedy marking a quick end? Both possibilities make me grasp each minute as precious. I acted more cautiously now, afraid I might speed things along by neglect or stupidity. I double-checked blind spots while driving, stepped carefully over curbs and down the stairs, focused when using a knife or power tool, and was vigilant with medical check-ups and self-care.

If I'm to live a long life, the day will come when my gait slows and requires a cane… to be replaced by a walker… and then a wheelchair. I will sell the house and Birdhouse to move into a two-room apartment on the main floor, then eventually a small room with a single hospital bed and a view of a tree from the window of someone else's home. When I cannot turn my head anymore to see the view, this scene, evening in the canyon, my years with Jack, will play inside my mind. Until then, I come to the Birdhouse to move my body, think, and remember.

To live on.

The setting sun illuminated only the top tenth of the surrounding eastern hills, like a row of golden berets. As time passed, the tallest, an actual mountain, was the last to say "Adieu" before the light and its beret were gone. The long shadows of the pines on the hillsides began to blend into the graying earth. I raised my cup of Irish coffee, its sweet steam of Baileys and Jameson rising through the whipped cream, and whispered, "Adiós," to these darkening eastern hills.

The evening sky turned into a navy-blue sea, and there in the southern sky was the first pinprick of light, "One" of twenty-one stars we once counted together, Sirius, in the Dog constellation, my only dog with me tonight.

Gone were Sneakers, Annie B, and Little Anna. For the third time in over thirty years, I was dogless; responsible for only myself. All the sounds in the house belonged to me. But that silence made the air feel brittle. Thin. I was living half a life without a dog in it.

I lacked the enthusiasm for the game of "21" stars tonight, so I went in around the seventh. Out through the windows, the land was blanketed in black. Turning on the lamp by my chair, I saw only my reflection in the glass and closed the blinds. I needn't be reminded.

When I arrived for this visit, I was startled as I opened the front door. The open room felt hollowed of the life it once held, like an abandoned seashell, only a shadow of someone who sat in that chair and slept in that bed. The sounds of laughter and love dusted all surfaces. The air was sweeter with Jack and Annie B here. I missed all that my old life contained; moments that I wanted back desperately, so desperately.

"I miss you guys so much," I said to the great room as I stepped onto the entry blue rug.

Then, up from the floorboards, through the gray industrial carpet, I heard their whispers, "We miss you, too."

Chapter 26
Swimming: Online Dating Experience

"What kind of woman in this world would see a close-up photo of a man holding a skunk next to his cheek and think, *I gotta meet this dude?*" I hollered at my computer screen on my first morning of online dating. On a reputable site, this man, in a black tank top, sporting an untrimmed woolly mustache and mop of hair, was posed with a skunk, not with a golden retriever or a Siamese cat. Even a bowl of goldfish would have been better. *Please tell me that's not his pet.* This man and I had nothing in common except that we were in the same fifty-to-seventy age bracket (I was sixty years old) and had paid the first-month fee of $60 to view other interested and available senior singles. Studying his profile, I was curious, but only about the skunk. *Oh, my God, what have I gotten myself into?*

Jack died five years ago. My heart was still anchored to him and always will be. A soulmate marriage, a best friend. I thought there was only one man like Jack in this world for me, and everyone else would be second best, but "second best" sounded better than another quiet week alone. Guilt simmered and radiated an accusation: *Cheater.*

Standing before the mirror in the bathroom, I spoke to my late husband. *But wouldn't I want the same for you, Jack, if circumstances were reversed?* At the kitchen counter, I picked up the conversation where it left off. *Live on, Jack. That's what I would say to you. Hug and love another.* Walking the dog, I added, *Life is short. Don't be alone unless you want to be.* Driving to the store, I made my closing argument. *After all, our marriage was supposed to be "until death do you part," and you did part on me, Jackson.*

I was ready for something new. I worked through the hard grief with my therapist and attended the widowed support group. I accepted my fifth-wheel status at friends' holiday meals and survived the empty car and house waiting for me afterward.

Women gave me friendship and company, but I also wanted what men offered: differing viewpoints on the world, even if they were sometimes goofy and illogical; an attitude of confidence that I envied; playful banter; and tenderness. I wanted meals out with a date, and an occupied seat next to mine at the theater, symphony, or lecture hall, even a simple tea or coffee hour. I craved someone asking me, "What did you do today?" and then hearing how he filled his day. A hand to slip around mine. Another dog lover. Not a husband. Just a male buddy, perhaps with "benefits." I won't lie, I missed good sex with a partner. But that could wait. I'd look for friendship first.

At the support group meeting one night, the speaker gave the following statistics: if a widowed man or woman entered their next marriage only one year after the death, ninety percent of those relationships would fail. At the two-year mark, the failure rate dropped to eighty percent, and with a ten percent drop each year thereafter until five years following the death, the chances of a lasting relationship were the same as the general population: fifty-fifty. Not optimistic odds, but better than my present "zero-zero." *Wait, heal, and don't rush to fill the void* were the keys before entering a new partnership.

This morning, at the weekly coffee gathering, a lull in the conversation was my opportunity to hop in with my news to the group. "I'm thinking of trying online dating." I tossed the confession onto the table like a poker chip in a card game. All conversation stopped, and my friends exchanged wide-eyed glances. A warm blush rose in my cheeks, and my mouth went dry.

I sipped some tea, thinking, *Do I sound like a slut? Did I misspeak and say something outrageous like, "I'm pregnant?"*

I was the first widow in this group of peers. What did they know of widowhood? Had they not listened all these years, or did I not adequately tell them of my loneliness? Did they only see the tough, determined, independent woman who endured it all?

After swallows of coffee and bites of scones and croissants, Denise cleared her throat, peered over her rimless glasses, and said, "Well, it's been a long time since Jack died. Why not?"

"I suppose so," Joyce said. "How long has it been?"

With raised eyebrows, Denise stuttered through her question. "But if you meet someone… and he dies first… are you willing to go through it all again… as you did with Jack?"

Behind that question, I heard, *Are you crazy?*

Maybe I was, but she was with her husband, and I was the one with a miniature Rat Terrier as my only companion. One recent weekend, I made several phone calls to see if anyone was free to go to a movie. At two homes, I was told, "No, we have plans," and at her home, "I'll have to ask John to see if we're doing anything." She only had to walk into the other room to find him. And he came first.

"I love my husband, but I can't wait to be alone," said another with a chuckle. She envied my single status and yearned for the day when she was not worn out by the peculiarities and demands of her aging spouse. He was a difficult man, not one I would have picked. I'm not sure if I would have survived with my sanity intact after decades in that marriage. Widowhood for her may well be easier than marriage.

Yes, of course, I imagined the pain of losing another love. But I already knew hell, and how to survive dying and death. How to live on. I met several widows in the support group whose second relationships ended with death, and they survived it. They inspired me. I believed my friends were trying to protect me from another loss and from the hassles of bringing a new man into my life. But what did they know of a widow's life on the weekend?

I did my research: recent studies found that one-third of all relationships started online. The eligible dates were limited: not colleagues from work (I am a retiree), not from church (a non-attendee), not the bar scene (fearful of clubbing or being clubbed), and not setups by friends (all their brothers and young uncles were already married).

Contrary to sage advice: *Meet people at places and events you enjoy*, trust me on this, the single men were not there. I tried. I didn't find single sixty-year-old men standing around in the lobbies of theaters or on the sidelines of co-ed adult soccer games. Maybe they were at hot rod shows or fishing and hunting exhibitions, but that would entail understanding carburetors, tying fishing flies, loading and shooting guns, and feigning interest for the remainder of the relationship. Maybe in the aisles on "Senior Discount Tuesdays" at a local grocery store, where some blocked the aisle with their slow gaits, in stretched-out cardigans and drab wrinkled pants, likely toting sad baskets full of single-serving cans of soup and loaves of white bread. The only solution I saw for a safe date for a youngish widow of the Baby Boomer generation was a senior online dating site.

I, too, was on the backside of this same hill of aging. Everything was slower and sagging on me. But I still had the wit and intelligence to be a fun date. Single men of similar energy and interests must be out there looking for someone like me. Would I warrant a turned head and once-over when I walked by? Tell me, where and when do they shop?

One Monday night, after another uneventful weekend, I became determined that the next weekend would be different. A teaching friend advised a student spinning in place with a problem, *Go to the solution.* On the couch, in sweatpants and an old soft flannel shirt, little Anna nestled into my hip, a Merlot uncorked, and the laptop booted up, I declared myself ready. I was in "go to solution" mode, taking the first step into the shallow end of the dating pool.

I studied the pros and cons of various sites and read reviews posted by users. Most reviews were over-the-top positive. I noted the lack of negative reviews and decided women who had terrible experiences with online dating sites had likely been reported missing to the local police. I read in the newspaper the horror stories about stalkers who could find you no matter where you hid. Panic began to cramp my typing fingers.

One site had safety walls that protected members from what I feared most (aside from abduction): the rude, crude, and vulgar. The site had an easy process for reporting bad behavior. All profiles were pre-approved and screened for improprieties and innuendos before they were made public, which soothed my jitters. Plus, the first swallows of wine had hit my head.

Still, I trusted no one, so I created my own structure for safety and peace of mind. Before opening the site, I created a new email address, essential for anonymity and protection of my home account. If I wanted communication to stop, all access to me would drop to the bottom of a cyber pit. I would give no one my full real name, personal email address, phone number, or home address. A face-to-face meeting would always be at a public place like a local café, mid-morning in a town twenty minutes from my home. I'd drive myself. I would drive away after he did, noting his car, stop at a store on the way home, and check my rearview mirror often.

Onto the dating site. Step One: my personal public profile, posted on the site for members to see. This required a long sip of wine. The profile entailed filling in personal parameters: age bracket, social drinker/not, children at home/not, work, income, religious preferences, hobbies, activities, favorite movie, TV show, and books, religion/or not, body type, smoker/non-smoker. After the most basic info was entered, the site asked questions to gauge compatibility.

"What would be a perfect first date?"

This question stopped me. It had been thirty years since I began to date Jack. I wanted to keep it simple while making it clear that the dog was part of the bargain. "Coffee or tea, and maybe a walk with the dog afterward." Another sip of wine. I was wading in, up to my shins in the pool.

"Who should pay for a meal?" Don't mind paying my half.

"How important is a sense of humor?" Very.

These answers would separate the desirable from the not-so-desirable. We would know something about each other before ever making contact. Great system, if everyone told the truth.

Step Two: My "tag," my online name, would attach to my profile page and be what men called me until I revealed my actual first name. I didn't want to use one word that sounded like a *Dear Abby* letter, "Lonely," "Anxious," or "Curious," especially when "Terrified" was more accurate. What would be inviting but not suggestive? Not

"HotGreyingMomma" or "CheapButNotEasy." I settled for an honest "Me&Dog&Life."

Step Three: Photos. Photos without Jack by my side were necessary. I'd had my picture taken only twice since Jack died. Once, while vacationing on the Oregon coast, I asked a stranger to take a photo so I could tease non-retired friends: "I'm playing, you're working." My body-shot photo showed me in shorts and a T-shirt, little Anna at my feet, with Oregon's Haystack Rock in the background. The second photo was on a departing ramp of a cruise ship, my arm over the shoulder of a woman friend. Cropping her out made an adequate headshot: a brunette with a short travel haircut.

Step Four: Payment. I needed a second glass of wine. I could close the laptop, lean back into the couch, scratch Anna's head, and find a Hallmark Channel movie. No one was forcing me to do this. But one of my personal mantras was, *If not now, when?* I got up and retrieved the credit card from the other room. Now. My heart thundered in my chest. I mistyped my credit card number three times before nailing it. I could handle $60 for one month, but a fear rattled through me: would someone out there be buying car tires and expensive jewelry on my card? I was nervous, but I was already in the pool, deep enough to know I wasn't getting out. Taking the final gulp, I shut the computer down at 10:30 p.m., thinking I'd wasted three hours of time and musing that my monthly fee would have bought a lot of good wine.

Waking up at an early 5:30 a.m., after a *What the hell have I done?* night of sleep, I rushed to my computer and checked for strange charges made to my credit card. None. Phew.

Friends experienced with online dating warned me that the busiest time for interaction was the first week, after which interest waned. I opened the dating site. HOLY SHIT! In those seven hours, over eighty men had checked my profile. I knew this because their tags and times of viewing were posted. I was fresh roadkill with a murder of crows flying overhead. What kind of guys examine profiles at three in the morning?

I learned the need to be specific with all the given filters, some of which I skipped last night, starting with the distance from home: a preferred thirty miles from Seattle as opposed to the entire United States. Men from Florida, Delaware, Wisconsin, California, and elsewhere had read my profile. Sitting at the dining table, aghast at what I'd gotten into, my hands shaking, a *Bing!* sounded from the computer, and a small box popped up: "Joe345 is looking at your profile." I clicked on his photo and then his profile. He was 59 (good) but lived in New York. After explaining to him my mistake of skipping the filters, I didn't want to appear rude, so my right pinkie hit the first "delete" of the day.

Another quick *Bing!* "LoveMyTractor is looking at your profile." As I opened his profile, one question shouted out from the photo: Where was the screening part of this program? I was an athletic college graduate with season tickets to live theater, and I saw a man in faded overalls and a red long-john shirt, standing in front of a quarter-moon cut-out on the door of what I assumed was an outhouse. Holding an 18" trout was not a selling point. I wrote "Dog lover" in my profile, not fish lover, not skunk lover. Was he dressed like this as a joke? Second delete.

The dating site was like Facebook on speed, like a Las Vegas casino with bells and whistles going off all the time. I pulled down any screen, and more options flashed in. Faces twirled across the screen like ponies on a carousel. An "Alert!" box informed me of missed "Who's looking at you?" notifications if I stepped away. Red heart icons smattered everywhere.

Based on how I answered the profile questions, the program sent out a high school yearbook-looking page with twelve to fifteen men as potential matches. I promised myself not to waste that $60, so I set my eyes on the deep end of this pool. I hopped through the photos (one man wore a Green Bay "Cheesehead" for his photo, cute), read their profiles for commonalities, selected a couple of potentials, and sent a "wink," which was like baiting a hook and tossing it back into the lake: bite or no bite? With some, I skipped the "winks" and jumped straight to emailing conversation openers: "I read on your profile that we have [this in common]." If I was in this pool, I was going to swim.

When meeting a future employer, an applicant has ten seconds to make a good impression. I, too, made quick judgments based on little information. What was initially a careful study, examining closely photos and reading everything in each profile, eventually became, after just a few hours on the site, a casual glance and skimming of words. Someone must tell some of these men that they were getting only two or three seconds with the photo and a fifteen-second scan of their profiles, if, a big IF, I clicked on their name.

"Put some effort into it," I yelled at the screen. "Try to impress me."

Men with dogs in their photos at least got a look. Some were single for an obvious reason. One of my deletes was the man who took a picture of his smile, just his smile, without photoshopping out the yellow teeth and receding gum line. Not that my teeth were any better, but I wouldn't put them out there as a selling point. Delete "Skunk with a Man," "LoveMyTractor," and "Smiley." Ten seconds, guys. Ten seconds at best.

With my morning tea and cereal on the dining room table, laptop open, my day started with "Who is looking at me?" Hours slipped away.

Throughout the day, between dog walks, the bing… bing… bing pulled me from chores and away from my meals to check on the men.

Up in the right-hand corner of the screen, boldly marked, was the total number of viewings plus an arrow on a barometer indicating various levels: "You're doing OK. Maybe contact more people?" or "You're being noticed." My little yellow arrow pointed to the top designation of the scale: "You're popular!" I was right back in high school, wondering if anyone would ask me to prom. Now I was the head cheerleader and not the real me, the dumpy, shy adolescent who never went to high school dances. "Popular" was never a word to describe me. What a hoot. I saw how addictive and seductive it was to keep that arrow on "Popular," but much like high school, I had no idea how to maintain this momentum.

The men I met at cafés recognized me immediately from my profile photos. I wanted the same. The profile choices for describing one's build were "Slim," "Athletic," "Average," "Heavy." *Bing!* My profile was being viewed by a man with the right age and education, matching me in many fields, but he selected "Average" for his build, while his photo clearly showed "Heavy." He could be on a terrific weight-loss program, or not, goal-oriented and a nice guy, but I didn't want to be surprised at a meet-up. Pitiful were those seniors whose photos showed themselves as twenty-something-year-olds in military uniforms. Or worse yet, the ones who used cartoon or comic book characters. Talk about a turn-off. I wanted honesty. Upfront. Now.

My stated interests and hobbies were really mine, not some feeble attempt to impress anyone. I expected that from men, too. I deleted what sounded like arrogance: "*I know what you women want.*" Obnoxious answers to the "Ideal First Date" profile question included, "After a candlelit dinner, let's walk on the beach with a glass of wine and read poetry together," and "Holding your hand while watching *Mama Mia* or *Little Women*." Delete and delete.

Besides my college education, I listed that I enjoyed reading books and was writing one. *Bing!* A nice-looking man popped up but sent the comment, "I only read the bible [his lack of capitalization] and service manuals." Hmm, those are similar genres, no? What would be the conversation if we chatted by email: "Is there a manual that is your favorite?" On the first face-to-face meeting, would I bring along my washing machine manual or, to be daring, the miter saw? In a similar vein, another man sent the message, "Don't read that much; I think I get enough reading the bills." Yet another listed two of his inspirational people as "Dolly Lama" and "Eckhart Toll." In fifteen seconds, the misspellings and grammatical errors doused any interest.

Unexpectedly, via the computer screen, I faced my judgments and prejudices with each click of that delete key. Clothing, hairstyles, backgrounds and foregrounds, activities, religious symbols, tattoos, weight, and height jumped out from pictures. I found that I did not "wink" at some men of color, or men shorter than my 5'5" (I was used to Jack's 5'10"), or those lacking post–high-school education, or men from cultures that limited women's rights. I found myself wondering, with a new self-awareness: was I no better than my parents, who always lived in all-white suburban neighborhoods?

"Bill, not in front of the children," Mother would admonish Dad when he told a demeaning racial joke or used a racial slur at the dinner table, but said it with a snicker in her voice. I heard it.

Those judgments, which I thought I had cleansed from my thinking, slithered out from my childhood, triggered by a photo or a few words in a profile. I wasn't any better than "Skunk-Man" or "LoveMyTractor." I was just subtler; I didn't speak my intolerances out loud. I presented myself as accepting and open to differences. But I used the delete key without anyone knowing why. I knew, and I was embarrassed at my lack of personal growth after sixty years of life.

Age was another can of worms. At a group luncheon months earlier, an eighty-year-old widower friend and I talked about dating. He warned me, "You will be a hot number with your pension. Be careful." His words whirled in my head when both older and younger men "waved" at me online. I skipped over those in their seventies and older, because I didn't want to be their "nurse with a purse." I'd buried Jack just five years ago, when he was only sixty. Although there was no guarantee of how many years were left in any life, my chance of a second widowhood was greater with older men. On the other hand, I wondered about men in their early fifties and what they saw in me. Only the "purse?"

"Will relocate," some wrote, "if I find the woman of my dreams." I translated this to: *I will move my trash into your house and freeload off you.* My cynical side wondered how many women in his community he'd burned by not paying half the rent, filling the refrigerator, or treating her to a meal out. How far would he travel to find anonymity in a new town? Stay put where you are, I murmured to the screen, and deleted.

Another profile category was marital status. Check one of the following:

- "Never married" (I clucked at one man, sixty-four years old, who had never married but was searching. Why now? Needing a nurse?)

  - "Divorced."

  - "Widowed."

- "Separated." (You're dating without a divorce?)

It was unbelievable to me that any man using the last available option would attract female interest: "Tell You Later." No, tell me right now, I demanded of the man on the screen. If you can't be honest and open, my gut says you lie about work and income, and you're probably a polygamist. Delete.

When I booted up the program on the third morning, I felt a soft vibration run from the keyboard into my fingertips. A hum of anticipation and hope radiated from the screen. *Maybe today I will meet him.* I saw in some men's words and eyes something I had missed. I knew this undertone because it sounded in my heart, too. The unspoken and honest reason we joined this site: loneliness. "To walk and talk together," "Travel to see new sights," "Make dinner together, sit on the couch, and watch old movies." This was what we wanted in one another. Not big events or dramatic activities. Not even marriage, but those everyday simple moments of being connected, touched, and remembered. One man nailed it, admitting, "I get tired of the mirror being the only reflection I see."

"Me, too," I cried at the computer screen. "Me, too." I sent him a "wink."

In ninety-six hours, I winked at twenty men, got eleven responses, continued chatting two or three times a day with six of those, reported one for profanity (the pseudo-Buddhist book reader fumed when I corrected his spelling), deleted fifteen, and passed my eyes over another fifty-two. Eventually, I met three for coffee and had second dates arranged for each. To balance it off, one obvious loser stood me up.

For four days, I savored the simple conversations among these single men. I learned to swim the breaststroke in this dating pool. I was less alone with these virtual friends; their wit had me leaning back in my chair with howls of laughter as they, in turn, laughed back at my Irish retorts. After five years without Jack, the cyber-warmth of male friendship rekindled what I was missing: simple daily conversations. The "Good morning. What are your plans today?" and "Good night. Sleep well. We'll talk tomorrow" gave me a familiar start and end to a day. Someone knew I was alive and wanted to talk to me. Others touched my heart with their sincerity, especially those dog lovers who invited my dog along for walks. I felt attractive; someone saw me as a friend. Hope radiated in my heart.

I was a different woman. When a man opted to email me, I felt singled out from the blur of faces on a busy city sidewalk. Maybe it was just my looks, but I had to believe it was more: my ability to speak my mind in words, to understand others, to show compassion and humor. I was special again. Jack was smiling, glad that his wife wasn't alone and crying for him.

Chapter 27
Almost There: Jack's Last Cabin Stay

"We're almost there," I sighed to the empty car seat. I eased down from the freeway, State Highway 2 speed, stopped at the light, took a left, and drove up the narrow, paved canyon road, shoulders of nothing but loose gravel and rusty barbed-wire fences. Small coveys of quail skittered across on their toothpick legs; some took flight. The summer sun climbed over the eastern tan hills, a brightness that demanded sunglasses; the heat later in the day would prompt seclusion in the air-conditioned cabin. Both my car and life slowed down in this rural part of the state, away from the horns, sirens, and congestion of the city. The evening skies would sparkle a different story, too: the faint stars that hid behind commercial lights would join the bright ones in the Milky Way.

From the car speakers, music on my iPod played warm yet sorrowful memories. "Sweet-bitter" was what I called them: Sweet was the joy of a good time, followed by the bitter realization that it's never to be repeated. He's gone. Little things carried me back; I sometimes wanted to stay longer in those moments, even sad ones, and hit "replay." Other times, I skipped by, I didn't want to go where the lyrics would take me.

The absence of Jack and Annie B was accentuated on trips to the cabin. *I wish you guys were here with me.* My eyes moistened. In the vacant passenger seat, I saw Annie B's short, shimmering black fur with patches of tan and white socks on Jack's lap.

"We're almost there."

Annie B's ears perked forward, and she sat up whenever one of us made the announcement at the stoplight. With soft whines, she pressed her nose on the window until it was rolled down. Regardless of weather, she hung her head out and gulped in the air as only a dog could, excited to run free from a leash. Jack and I laughed, and I swore Annie B giggled too, with a sense of pure joy.

When Jack was healthy and both of us were working, the drive to the cabin gave us time to shift gears from the long, busy hours we spent apart as educators in two different schools into what we called "509 time," a reference to the area code for the eastern side of the state, where life seemed simpler and slower. We spent our drive engaged in conversation, catching each other up, "News Broadcasting," as we called it, which invariably started with, "I didn't tell you about what happened two days ago with this parent..." Jack would listen, maybe ask a question, but wasn't obligated to respond. When I was done, he'd begin a totally unrelated story: "Last night's wrestling match was a tough one..." We bounced back and forth with short snippets from our week, or even weeks before, until both of us became silent. All caught up. Ready for "509 time."

"We're almost there."

Annie B was always on my lap when Jack drove. She shifted over to his lap when his deteriorating health and pain meds took him out of the driver's seat. Annie B kept her front seat spot on his lap until the final month of Jack's life; anything pressing against his chest aggravated the cancer pain. She was relegated to the back seat. We also stopped "News Broadcasting"." Jack slept most of the way. I had so much to tell him. *So, this will be how it will be driving when he is gone, this god-awful silence.*

During what would be our last stay at the Birdhouse in early June, three weeks before his passing, we kept to our travel routine. After leaving Bellevue, the first "pit stop" was in Cle Elum, seventy minutes away, where Jack stirred enough to whisper, "I don't have to go." After my own relief, I walked the dog and worried that Jack wasn't getting enough fluids. Twenty minutes later, up Blewett Pass, amidst the jagged canyon walls, mountains, and tall evergreen, alder, and cedar trees, we stopped at a small espresso stand. He didn't order the usual blended mocha, like I did, but an orange smoothie. An orange smoothie? I watched him take one sip, put it back in the cup holder, and return to sleep.

At the Birdhouse, I said to Jack, "I'll unpack the car. You go take a nap."

"Good idea," he said wearily. He leaned on me as I guided him up the three stairs to the front door and to the bed, where he sat, and I took off his shoes.

"Anything to drink? Hungry? Gotta go to the bathroom? Warm enough? Want a blanket?" I rattled off the well-used questions and paused after each one for an answer. Most days, the bulk of our conversation hinged on these inquiries.

"No, nothing," he said, and then his eyes were closed again.

After the luggage, cooler, and food bags were inside, the last item to bring in was the smoothie. I walked to the kitchen, pulled out the straw, and tossed it in the garbage bin. A fine dust covered the kitchen windowsill, a dust carried by the northern wind that somehow found its way into the house through closed windows. With my index finger, I drew a line through it and wiped the residue onto my shorts. A chore for later: vacuum the sills, I thought. No, not vacuum, I corrected myself, as Jack would be sleeping most of the time. Use a moist rag.

Through the window, I watched the dark maroon leaves of the fifteen-foot-high maple tree out back and noted the empty suet holder and hummingbird feeder. Another chore. We planted the small sapling several years ago, a gift from Jack's staff as a memorial to his sister who died of cancer. I can't remember what kind of cancer. Jack would've known, but I didn't ask; it felt awkward, wrong, to talk with him about someone, especially family, who died from cancer. A covey sneaked out from under the wild roses into the clearing near the tree, and they pecked at the ground. *Got to toss seed out there,* I thought. Later.

The chill in my hand, the smoothie, brought my attention back to why I came into the kitchen. I poured the melting drink, along with any hope that this trip would energize Jack, down the drain.

Jack went to bed earlier, slept longer, and got up late each morning on this two-day stay. His head was shaved a month ago after the radiation for the brain tumors. Now he had only a gray stubble crown. His gray mustache stayed intact this time, unlike last year when he had the chemo. He was so thin: his clothes seemed to drip like candle wax off his once-muscular body. He dressed in a T-shirt under his long-sleeve Henley and sweatpants on a warm late spring day, while I wished for the air conditioner to be turned on. He ate little of his favorites I prepared. Less conversation, smaller meals. No lovemaking.

This stay was a hideous glimpse into my future. I detested the stillness; the quiet chafed against my skin. I wanted to yell, *Fight it, Jack, fight it. Get up!* But I didn't. He was a tired boxer who had fought long and hard. He deserved to rest.

Fuck you, Cancer, fuck you! I mouthed quietly. I held my fists at my sides when I wanted to punch a wall. *Fuck it all!*

After I checked in on Jack, listening to the purring of his breath, I went out. Standing on the deck in the sunlight, I surveyed the acreage. Someday, all the maintenance and repair of the Birdhouse would be mine. Most of it was straightforward and doable, I could manage, but major repairs, without Jack's skills, would involve hiring someone reliable. A woman alone in need of a reliable person, in a man's domain of plumbing, roofing, and electrical. My throat tightened, and I swallowed down panic.

Just here, just now, I reminded myself. I could not worry about future breakdowns when I had enough to do with Jack inside.

The tractor was the essential key piece of equipment for heavy and hard work made easier, and I knew nothing about it. Like so many of our remodeling projects, which involved new skills, me as an eager student, and Jack as teacher: drywall, roofing, installation, plumbing, electrical, I needed lessons on "Boomer," the tractor.

Up from his hour nap, Jack rode Boomer for a few swaths through the front grass, then stopped, too tired to finish the two-hour job. I watched him struggle for balance as he stepped off the seat to the ground, muscle atrophy making his movements slow and wobbly. I grabbed a glass of water from the kitchen and rushed to him, so he had me for balance. He took a few sips, returned the glass to me, and leaned against the tractor.

I began to ask about the basics: How do you start it? Which way does the lever move to lower and raise the bucket? How do you engage the mower?

Jack stared at the tractor. With a long sigh, he said to the ground, "I should have gotten you on the tractor more." His voice cracked.

"No," I snapped, and stepped in front of him to look into his watery eyes. "It's your tractor and your job. I never wanted one second on it."

We bought Boomer when Jack first got his diagnosis four years ago, to replace an aging used tractor that we had bought off a neighbor. I had hoped the new machine would give him joy and, as crazy as this sounds, boost his immune system with the fun he had riding it. Anything to extend his life, or, at worst, provide something he enjoyed in his final days.

Diverting my gaze to the horizon, I added softly, "I will have time later."

I brought my eyes up to meet his, and we both cried as I fell into his chest, his arms around my shoulders and mine around his slender waist. I felt a soft kiss on the top of my head before he unwrapped his arms.

"Go, get up on it," Jack said, one hand waving toward the seat while the other wiped his eyes. I wanted to fight him, but the murmur in my head warned, "This is his last visit to the Birdhouse. It's now or never." I needed Boomer to maintain this place.

Jack pointed to the key and explained the clutch and brake pedals. I started it. He placed a hand on the lever to raise and lower the bucket.

"Put everything in neutral, but keep it running," he said. I did.

"See this knob?" I nodded. "It engages the PTO, which engages the mower." I nodded again, although I had no idea what a "PTO" was. But I knew by his fading voice there wasn't time for more questions.

He leaned into a garden fence post for balance as I engaged the mower and mowed twenty or so yards, drove into its storage area, disengaged the PTO, released the bucket and mower to the ground, and turned off the engine with an "I did it. That's good enough." Jack said, "Good job," with the weariness of a man who had walked miles in the hot sun. I walked over to him, ducked under his arm, and with my hand around his waist, we shuffled back inside to the bedroom. Naptime for Jack. Once he was asleep, I went out into the vegetable garden and wept.

I did eventually learn how to use the tractor beyond the basics Jack showed me that day. I studied the manual and asked questions of my neighbor, Kermit, and a man at the repair shop in town, though most of the learning was by trial and error. I mowed too low and clipped rocks; mowed too high and missed the tall grass and weeds altogether. I loaded cuttings into the bucket but watched the poorly stacked contents fall along the path to the burn pile. The mower nicked the corners of the woodshed and bricks along the graveled front when I misjudged how much space was needed for turns. I almost backed over an edge that would have sent the tractor and me tumbling down ten feet. Wisely, I always wore the seat belt. With each mishap, I cried to the heavens, "Help me, Jack!" then sighed, "Thanks, Bud, that could have been bad."

After Jack's death, Annie B returned to the passenger seat with its new creamy-yellow lamb's-wool fleece for her aging bones. She slept most of the way, like Jack in his final months, but I wasn't alone. Her old body was slow to rise when I announced, "We're almost there," at the turn, but she still wanted the window down. In another year, I will put her to rest.

After nine months of being dogless, I adopted an elderly rescue dog, Anna. Anna was ten years old when I met her, a Rat Terrier with medical issues, and I was her fifth owner. She was loving, house-trained, and a good traveler. Summers at the Birdhouse, she was also anxious to get out of the car to smell the honey scent of dried warm grass that filled the air. In winter, she gave me the Rat Terrier bug-eyed look of "*Pick me up now!*" when the snow was too deep for her ten-pound body to traverse. She had Addison's disease and was doomed to either organ failure or a stroke. Indeed, after only thirty-eight months together, I had her put to rest after a major stroke.

Three months after Anna's end, a pair of Chihuahua-mix rescues, Hope and Penny, became my traveling companions. Regardless of the dog in the car, and there will always be one or two, when I steered up the canyon road, I missed Annie B the most. The passenger side of the car was still designated as her side. I sometimes rolled down the window so the dry air filled the car. From the corner of my eye, I saw her head hanging out the open window, a tradition as much a part of the trip as packing food and a toothbrush.

And I said to the breeze, "We're almost there."

Upon arrival at the Birdhouse, I got out and went around to the back car door to lift out "the girls" from their travel crate. They dashed from the garage to sniff the evidence of deer, rabbits, and neighbors' dogs who'd trespassed on the four acres of land in their absence, found snacks in the wildlife droppings, startled the quail from the thorny wild rose bushes, and emptied their bladders after the two-and-a-half-hour trip.

Out of the two-car garage Jack and I built as an addition onto the small modular home, I walked several yards toward the corner of an L-shaped retaining wall. The adobe-colored block wall was installed a few months after Jack's passing, my first autumn as a widow. I remember staring at the samples at the mason supply company, feeling the empty space in my head where his second opinion should be. My heartbeat drummed at my temples: I was making a several-hundred-dollar decision. So unlike paint, if I picked the wrong color, I could simply cover it up with a new hue. The block wall would be four feet high, six rows of blocks, and seventy-five feet long. An expensive mistake if I chose wrong. Permanent. I would look at this for the rest of my life at the cabin. Although Jack usually seconded my selection of décor designs and colors, I began to question my choices after his passing. Where did my confidence go? I rattled a prayer from my heart: *"Oh, Bubba, ya gotta help me here."* But I didn't hear his choice that day.

The block wall was yet another expense that chewed at the life-insurance check in my savings account. Another "Gotta get this done immediately" task: the winter rain and snow would collapse the piles of soil meant for filler. It would be another spring backhoe/dozer job, another check to write, if I waited until the snow melted. I also had to find the labor to build the "L"-shaped wall with those twenty-four-pound blocks. It was our garage that we built together, but I managed the completion of the project alone.

Every visit, I walked across the compressed gray gravel and stopped at the corner L. I brought two fingers to my lips and, leaning over, placed the kiss on the gray block three from the bottom, behind which lay a third of Jack's ashes, with "I miss you, Bud," or "Bubba," "Jack," "Jackson," or "JR," whichever endearment fit my heart that day. The sandpaper texture was rough on my fingertips, much like Jack's two-day stubble. I kissed my fingers again and tapped the gray block two above Jack's, where Annie B's ashes were. "I miss you too, Booff," "Ms. B," "Annie," or "B." I wanted to hear back, "I miss you too, Talle," or "Bubbett," or "Baby Butts," but I heard only the northern wind whoosh through the trees.

Two gray blocks among the adobes. I knew where they were. I was not alone.

I survived the worst of widowhood in those first five years, maintained the land and houses here and there. I sat on the wood bench we put together from a kit, which I repaired this season, on the deck we built. After a long day of gardening and maintenance chores, I showered, ate whatever I brought for dinner, and sat myself here, wondering how many more years I could keep this pace up. With two glasses, one red wine and the other water, with only Hope by my side, Penny had already curled under the bed sheets. I watched the sunlight dim.

After Jack's passing, Ralph, his dad, told me that I needed to find a "Grandfather who wants to putz around" for the small jobs and repairs around the cabin. "There will just be too many to do. It will wear you out." I asked around town. No one has stepped up for the role. Each season has its list of "to-dos" that must get done. If I don't do it, I only foresee a much larger repair bill looming seasons later for the neglect. Up the one-story roof I go to tighten the green metal roofing screws, clean the air vents of wasp nests, and brush the ash in the smokestack. Into the three-foot-high crawlspace to attach the heating coil to the water pipe from the well to prevent the pipe from freezing. Caulking dried siding seams, dried out from years of extreme temperatures. The tractor needed a full tank of diesel and a gas additive, and a battery taken out and hooked up to a trickle for winter storage. Letting a battery die was expensive; I replaced two already. I can't keep the place unless I am willing to keep up the maintenance.

If only someone would take me on that drive and roll down a window for me, so I could hang out my head, suck in hope from the warm country air, and hear them say, "We're almost there."

Chapter 28
[Poem]

Waiting

The loss of long days

and warm nights deepens

the chill. Nature retreats, turns

within.

Dying and death

are on the barren limbs,

in the sleeping garden. Fallen

remnants of what was once grand

now spattered and decaying.

Beneath the frosted ground,

crocus and tulips rest.

The hope of spring

awaits. The early warmth

of a winter day deceives

some to peek out of the ground

early. Burial and resurrection

have an order and a time.

Those fooled

will not see

the spring, only to die

in the returning bitter cold.

That, too, follows

an order. Even those who remain

in the dark do not always

bloom

in the spring.

They wither in the earth, weak,

or diseased, not strong enough to endure

the harsh season.

All are planted

with the hope of blooming a

new life

in the old soil.

So it is also

with grief and the grieving.

Chapter 29
Gifts: The Woman in the Mirror

In the soft light of a cloudy Northwest morning, in a bathroom scented with lavender soap and lotion, I study the woman in the mirror. She has the same coffee-colored eyes that gazed back in her old home's mirror, the one she shared with Jack. Irish wit and intellect spark within those eyes. But, five years since his death, these pools appear calmer, two still ponds. They are no longer outlined by swollen red lids or sorrow that brimmed to the edges, although some tears trickle out occasionally, on birthdays, anniversaries, and funerals. The snowy whites of her eyes have returned, surrounded by more crinkly lines than before: some grown from stress and fear, but others caused by smiling. Her shoulders and head no longer droop, so she can see beyond her shadow to the horizon. She is a warrior.

Until my own death, I will wear what I call "the tattoos of widowhood," marks that permeate beyond my skin into my marrow. With time, the ink fades, along with the details of those early years. My memories of the harshest struggles are softened. But when I hear stories from the newly widowed, my heart sighs, "*Oh, I remember that well.*"

I know to ask, "How did they die?"

"What did you do with his clothes? The ones in drawers and closets? Those dirty items in the laundry basket?"

"Tell me about the paperwork afterward: bills, car titles, I know there are so many pieces bearing the other's name and demanding your time."

"How do you handle the evenings alone? The bed?"

Their eyes will moisten. Their stories must be told dozens of times, over and over, until pain is squeezed out like water from a sponge. I know how to offer silence, softened eyes, a gentle lean toward the griever that says, "I know mine. I want to hear yours."

Now my own painful moments are kept in a battered box, like old receipts: the lost sleep, the loss of friends who never called or visited, moving his possessions, changing or dropping family rituals. Although the box seems full, there is room for more. I know how to hold onto the past and let go: shards of a shattered vase cannot be shaped into something new.

The indecisiveness and uncertainty, *I'm not as sure who I am anymore without Jack,* have been left by the wayside after five years. I learned to weigh those pros and cons and make my move. Those lonely, big decisions started on the day I chose which urn, where to bury his ashes, and when to hold his Celebration of Life. I learned what things I could do alone and those I could not.

When it came to furniture colors and styles, I asked for help from a talented home décor specialist. Paint-store clerks explained how to undo the walls' ugly hues. A window-covering specialist helped replace the metal blinds.

Thousands of other decisions were mine. Which dog to adopt? What's for dinner tonight? Which bulbs for the garden? I winterized and spring-readied the cabin, eventually referring to a typed list of necessary chores, created after years of *"Oops, forgot to do that."* Lists were vital. I hired someone to mow the acres twice a month during spring and summer, which gave me time to do simple repairs and maintain the vegetable garden for the late-summer harvest, shared with friends and food banks.

In recent years, I rarely ask the heavens, "What do you think I should do, Jackson?" And if I do, it's more out of habit than seeking an answer. Jackson is quiet now. There are no dreams or visits. But in the soft breeze, when a dragonfly flies low in the yard, I feel his affirmation: "*You know what to do. Do it.*"

His last clear message came three years after his passing, while I washed and detailed "Max," his truck's nickname. The expense of keeping two vehicles, my Baja truck and Jack's Ford Ranger, had become illogical. I used his truck for three or four errands a year; license tabs and oil changes were more expensive than a one-day rental. Besides, neighbors had trucks I could borrow. A kind neighbor down the street had a used-car business and offered to sell Max for me, which would save me from dealing with strangers wanting test drives and bickering about price. I trusted him, and he promised more profit in my pocket than his.

But it's Jack's truck. It's Max! my heart screamed.

I recalled our many rides in Max, carrying various loads, bags of concrete, lumber, drywall, Christmas trees, a garage-sale lamp, and a sofa for the cabin, dirt for our garden beds. I had Annie B on my lap and watched Jack's chiseled profile as he drove. Full of happy memories, I second-guessed myself about selling Max. In the middle of the night, in the dark, I turned to the empty half of the bed and asked, "Tell me what to do, Jack."

On the day I was scheduled to drive Max over to the car lot, I vacuumed and washed the truck inside and out, scrubbed tires and rims, and cleaned every window. I began to wax Max's white body and chrome bumpers. This task kept my mind focused and my heart quiet until I found myself on my knees by the back bumper, no longer able to dam the tearful doubts that raced down my cheeks.

It's your truck, Bubba. Should I sell Max or not? Oh, Jackson, damn it, I need you here.

With that, his voice was suddenly behind me: "If it's the wrong decision, you know how to fix it."

I froze. My heart pounded and my eyes opened wide. *He's back!* I replayed his words, the sound of his voice. *He's back!* Did I really hear that? Was he kneeling behind me so that when I turned, I would see him, even if only as a faint image? I knew from other experiences that if I looked, he'd be gone.

Don't look, Tally, don't look. He might say more.

Crouched in the middle of the driveway, I had so many questions for Jack: about cabin maintenance, my finances, all the big and small decisions. How is heaven? How's Mom, Dad, your sister, Sneakers, and Annie B?

More than anything, I desperately craved to hear, "I adore you" one more time. "*Stay, please, stay,*" I thought, my eyes closed, praying for a few more words.

But that was all he said. I was alone again. His wisdom echoed in my head: his confidence in me silenced that critical voice that rants, "*You will muck things up.*" He was right; I knew what to do to fix a poor decision. God knows I'd done it enough times already.

Please be there, please be there. I slowly turned my head. Nothing.

The woman I see in the mirror today stands erect, with fewer hesitations in her expression. She sold a house, bought another, and dealt with mortgage companies, banks, and contractors. She traveled the world and took in new customs, sights, and colors. She skydived for her sixtieth birthday to continue the treasured tradition of birthday adventures she had with Jack and to embrace something entirely her own: the thrill of being on the edge. She held a powerful mantra: *Die with the fewest regrets.*

I expect to eventually lose height from the natural shrinking of the spine that comes with aging. I also know the aggravation of lifting those heavy moving boxes by myself, out from the old house into the truck, from the truck into the storage unit, out of the storage unit into a rental truck, and finally from the rental truck into this new house (thank God I had some help unloading), and then from room to room as I painted and unpacked, would likely impact my spine. Add the two dozen 24-pound retaining-wall bricks for the garden, loaded by the yard attendant at the garden center, but placed into a wall by me. And the six yards of topsoil I unloaded to expand the garden. I smile at how the yard looks so much better, fuller with blossoms almost year-round. Do the smiles from the tulips and irises help the back discomfort? I hope so.

I still climb up the ladder onto the two-story roof to blow off leaves, check seals on vents, scrape off moss, and clean the solar tubes. Someday, my back and knees will yell, "*Quit being so cheap and pay someone younger to do that chore!*" On that day, I will surrender a slice of my independence, no longer able to get a task done when it fits my schedule. I will find the patience to wait for a service truck to arrive and trust a stranger to get the work done. Until then, I climb up and down the ladder and check off another season of completed chores.

Whenever I am at the doctor's office, standing on the scale while the nurse presses the top of the metal ruler onto my head, I meditate on silly thoughts: *Tall, think TALL,* and tell the disks of my spine, *Decompress. STRETCH!* I'm relieved when 5'5" is recorded on my chart. Grinning, I step away, but someday the number will change.

In the first few months after Jack's death, the full-length mirror in our old house showed a different body. Already at an ideal weight, ten pounds slipped off and alarmed close friends. The next five pounds scared even me. That first summer allowed me to live in baggy elastic-band shorts and loose T-shirts, and winter in sweatpants, long-sleeve tees, and hoodies. When I wore dress pants to go out, the old ones billowed like sails, and I cinched my belts to unused holes. My cheekbones were more pronounced, arm and thigh muscles sharply defined, and hipbones protruded. As a health teacher and counselor, I knew the downward spiral of anorexia and its destructive damage to the body.

I needed to recover the appetite that had left when Jack no longer joined me at the table. I needed to swallow more vegetables, fruits, and proteins, something other than popcorn. Eating alone at restaurants was a no-can-do. I admired widows who talked at support meetings about reading books or working crossword puzzles in front of empty chairs. Trying to chew and swallow sorrow would trigger a gag reflex if I ate alone. Eating at our favorite places, like the local pho place, Lil Jon's cinnamon rolls, and 12th Ave Café buckwheat pancakes, would require me to answer the regular servers asking, "Can I get you anything else?"

Yes, I would think. *A healthy Jack sitting in that chair across from me.*

On a break from gardening one afternoon, a few weeks after Jack passed, I wanted an ice-cream blended drink at the local Baskin-Robbins. This was a spot Jack and I often visited and one that I had avoided entering in recent days, stopped by survivor's guilt: I could eat ice cream, and he could not. It was irrational, and that guilt kept me away from enjoying the foods we had loved together. On this day, I just wanted that ice-cream drink, a lunch with no nutritional value except some calories, some fat, a bit of calcium, and protein.

The cool air of the shop was a welcome contrast to the hot, breezeless summer day in the yard and sent shivers up my back as my sweat chilled. I was hoping for a high-school employee, someone who didn't know me, didn't know us. Instead, I stood before the very familiar co-owner, a middle-aged Asian woman whose accent told of her courage to travel to the U.S., learn to speak English well, and ultimately buy a franchise with her husband.

"I would like a medium mocha blast with the espresso and cream, please." She wouldn't even ask about the cinnamon, a given, or the whipped cream on top, which was only for Sundays when we splurged for that extra sweetness and comfort. It wasn't Sunday.

Don't ask about Jack, please don't ask about Jack. My eyes dropped to the tubs of ice cream inside the glass case near me.

"I know, I know your order," her soft voice sparkled. I looked up to see her turn to get the ice cream scoop and the blender jar, and she walked to where my favorite ice cream was. Over her shoulder, she called, "What? No husband today?"

A cold fog filled my head. My focus went back to the colorful tubs, plain vanilla, chocolate chip mint, cherry jubilee, rocky road, colors that began to wash together like watercolors. Her eyes went from the ice cream scoop back to me. If my T-shirt said, "Newly Widowed," would I be saved an explanation and be left alone?

Oh, God, help me. Jackson. Damn it, damn you, you should be here.

She stood still, waiting for my response.

I swallowed hard and wished I could lie, *Oh, he's visiting his dad in Spokane,* or *He's got a cold and is home watching baseball.*

My feet were planted on that vinyl floor while the rest of me felt like a willow in a strong wind, thin branches that swayed and bowed, nearly breaking. *Float away, float away.*

Her eyes remained on me. I could not lie.

"He"..."

That one phrase, the one that slices through denial into reality, that slaps a label on the event and why I was here alone, was stuck on the roof of my mouth. Licking my lips, I focused my eyes on the counter.

"He... passed away a couple of weeks ago."

Her eyes widened, and she said, "I am so, so sorry. He was a very nice man."

She turned away to blend the drink. Through the whirl of the blender, I replied, "Yes, he is," and felt the present tense slap the side of my head. Yes, he should be next to me, or home watching baseball, waiting for me to bring his same-as-mine drink home. I knew "is" was wrong, but I wasn't ready for "was." I wanted to leave without the drink, dart to my car, roll the windows up, and cry, but I wanted the drink, a small treat in what felt like a harsh and unfair world. To hold a small sliver of what was once ours.

I laid a twenty-dollar bill on the counter when she handed me the plastic cup and a straw.

Shaking her head, she said, "No, no. On me," and pushed the money back toward me.

"No, Jack would want me to leave a big tip. Please take it." I grabbed the drink and walked toward the door, not giving her a chance to say or do anything more.

I felt her eyes on the back of my head as I left her store. She had only ice cream and a few words of comfort to give. That was enough. The fog lifted a bit. I could see my car in the parking lot, and I headed to safety. The next time I wanted a blended ice-cream drink, I drove by to see who was serving at the counter. I learned to protect my heart.

I liked the trimmer appearance, what felt like being in a younger-appearing body, after the weight loss. I walked with the illusion that someone might look back at me and think, "Nice ass," now that there wasn't so much to jiggle.

But I didn't know how much this woman's body had changed until an evening dress was required attire for my first European cruise trip, fifteen months after Jack left this earth. I was a poor shopper, unable to meander through racks and pull separates into impressive ensembles. Unlike my little sister, Beth, who could create elegant Nordstrom-quality outfits with Goodwill throwaways, I often bought whatever was on the store mannequins. I had to see the color and combinations, and only then could I tell if it was my style or not.

I roamed aimlessly through the jungle of dresses. Some were too frilly, with lace wrapped around the neckline, too high-school prom, backless with spaghetti straps; or too matronly, with only my head and hands showing. Trying on a half dozen styles and colors, I shook my head at my reflection each time. Gawd awful. After four stores, impatience screeched inside my head: *This is stupid. Quit. Go home.*

Help arrived at the last store in the mall, and I surrendered to my ineptitude.

"What size are you?" the clerk asked, after listening to what I needed. I watched her eyes flick a quick head-to-toe assessment. While we were about the same age, she was dressed like a corporate manager in a tailored gray suit, white blouse, and a colorful scarf. I was in shorts, a polo, and running shoes. My cheeks reddened as I didn't look the part of an experienced traveler who was merely adding a new item to an already well-traveled wardrobe.

"Between an eight and ten, I think," I replied. I was befuddled. Two years ago, that would have been the right answer. But that day, I simply didn't know. How does one not know their size?

"No, you're a six," she said, her voice authoritative from years of sizing women up, and off she went for dresses while I waited in the dressing room.

No, I'm not a six, I thought as I watched her walk away. Beth, five years younger than I, was a size four or six. Since infancy, we had never been the same size, except for an occasional coat. Never pants or dresses. I had always been one or two sizes up from her, with wider hips and shoulders, smaller breasts, and two inches of height.

I would placate this clerk. She'd see her mistake, I thought, when zippers wouldn't budge past my hips or buttons didn't reach their holes across my chest, and she'd go back for eights. Maybe tens. I would hide my "I told you so" behind a smirk.

I was a six.

The mirror reflected that truth with the first black dress: an elegant, sleeveless dress with a cowl collar, just low enough in front to show a breastbone cleavage and hitting two inches above the knee. It was perfect. The reflection fought with who I had pictured myself to be for fifty-seven years: an ordinary, muscular, athletic, small-breasted woman whom only one man could ever love. I had been lucky enough to find him when I was twenty-seven. No one else could ever see me as funny, smart, caring, passionate, or beautiful again.

I missed Jack's amorous leers when we dressed together, his eyes that flashed, "I want you." Getting ready for an afternoon matinee, our theater outfits laid out on the bed, the whiff of freshly showered bodies melding with our individual scents, his lime aftershave and my own cologne. Brushing a soft hand on my legs, breast, or back as he walked by, he would coo, "Hmm, baby, you be looking good." I missed that feeling of being attractive, sexy, vibrant, in the eyes of another. No one would find me as sexy as Jack did, or so I'd always assumed. But my new reflection in the mirror begged to differ.

One of my favorite childhood stories was *Alice Through the Looking-Glass*. The story delighted my imagination, and my ten-year-old fingers poked at various spots in the large rectangle mirror in the family living room, waiting for the magical moment when my hand would ripple through the mirror and glide me into the world behind it. I slouched on the couch with disappointment when I could not get through that hard, cold surface.

Now I was there again, in front of a dressing-room mirror in a smartly fashioned cocktail dress. I asked the image of the woman I saw, *"How did you get here?"* She simply smiled at me through the glass.

Some gifts of life are not wrapped in holiday tissue, tied brightly with ribbons and bows, or received with a heartfelt "Why, thank you for your thoughtfulness." Like opening Pandora's box, these ill-timed "gifts" following illness, accidents, failures, and losses are life changers. No human will ever be the same once they remove the lid.

I know this because I've changed. I came to terms with surviving Jack's dying and death, and my widowhood. Lately, the darkening skies of evening and the dateless weekends do not warrant a full-blown pity party, but merely a pause—time to catch my breath, slow my heart, and accept the quiet house as my new normal. I limit myself to one glass of red wine, not the three glasses I once needed to numb the pain. I now have the focus to read entire books.

In the bathroom mirror, I see impermanence. Limited, precious time. Jack's death brought awareness of my own mortality. Will I die alone or be found by a neighbor and transported to a hospital room, where I will wake up in an empty room, confused? Will it be a slow death, with time to put things in order, or a quick, unexpected one, like a brain aneurysm or massive heart attack? Will I be aware of the decline from dementia and act before it's too late? Who will get my possessions, house, car, and cabin? Most importantly, who will take care of my dog? The will I made doesn't answer all these questions, nor silence the worries in the dark.

But today I have acceptance. This is my life. Just me, a single, mortal woman with a dog and a simple life.

Turning away from the bathroom mirror, I stopped midstride. I looked over my shoulder, right into her eyes, and said, "I love who you are. Ya done did good, girl. And, by the way," I winked, "nice ass."

Chapter 30
Lessons: What I Learned After Five Years

After Jack's last breath, I was certain that my own death, soon after his, would have been a blessing. Save me from the screams to the heavens, "Why him? Why now?" Stop the loneliness that filled my chest. Blind me from seeing the shining shards of my twenty-six-year marriage scattered at my feet. Indeed, my death would have been a gift, or so I thought.

But I lived on.

I lived on and learned my life had greater meaning than I ever thought possible, that the depth of my strength and courage knew no bounds. Eventually, I stood inside an empty house without collapsing into sorrow on the floor. Most remarkable and unexpected was the grin that returned to my face, blossoming into rejuvenating laughter.

This evolution took more than five years, with the guidance of a good therapist, supportive friends and family, and a determination to find my own answer to the question, "Why me?" What I learned is: I have a new purpose, to stand by other grievers, listen to the stories that churn inside their hearts and minds, and simply answer their questions with, "Me too. I remember something like that. It's common. It's universal. You're not crazy. You're not alone."

Lesson # 1: The Other Death Is Not Better

Some of my friends who have naturally straight hair envy those with natural curls. They seek salon perms to add wave to their straight tresses, as I once did. In contrast, my curly-haired friends sometimes wish for straight hair that wouldn't frizz up with humidity. Each type of hair has its challenges. The same illogical envy, I want what they have, exists between those who lost a loved one to a slow death and those whose loss was quick and unexpected. The fact is, no one had it worse; the other death is not better.

From diagnosis to his last breath, Jack's death took four-and-a-half years. I have straight hair. A soccer teammate's husband died unexpectedly on the operating table during a simple, routine procedure. A dear friend's husband had a massive heart attack during a nap while she was out of the house. Both have said to me, "You were so lucky to have that time with him. I never got to say goodbye." They have curly hair. While they wanted more time, I wanted less, especially at the end: I wished for Jack's suffering to cease. They assumed our last years together were filled with words of closure and grand declarations of love. They missed out on that. But in our first two years with cancer, we waited quietly between scans and blood tests, in the aftermath of surgeries, praying separately for tumors to shrink, that no new ones would be found, and for enough white blood cells to continue treatment. We hardly spoke of cancer, fearful that our words would crack the walls of denial we had built around ourselves. We pretended this cancer was beatable. Even in his two five-month remissions, never longer than that, cancer and death lingered silently in the shadows.

The last months of Jack's life were awful: I watched him slowly dissolve into someone who didn't give me the loving words I wanted to hear, much less speak of his own dying or death. I heard only "Yeah" or "No" in response to my, "Do you want some water? Jell-O? Gotta go to the bathroom?" My strong husband, a former athlete, dissolved before my eyes. Regardless of my efforts, I could not release him from death's grip and mold him back into his old self, my dear best friend.

A quick heart attack would have been a gift of mercy and love from my God. Desperately, in those last two months, I wanted curly hair.

This metaphor applies to the number of years each widow or widower had with their spouse, too. I attended a widowed support group and listened with envy to those silver-haired grievers who had celebrated their golden fiftieth anniversaries, or at least wore the pearls of their thirtieth. How I wanted more time, more stories to bob me up from the lonely depths. I got a little over twenty-six years old. But which was better, which was worse: more jabs at the heart from more pictures, artifacts, and memories that would constantly remind them of what once was? Or fewer, like me? What about that woman who was only married fourteen years before she lost her husband to a car accident? Does she envy me?

I had straight hair. The other death is not better.

Lesson #2: It's Okay to Have No Idea What You Did Today

In the early days of "the afterward," my friends often questioned, "What are you doing with your days?"

Some days were longer and harder than others in that first year. I had no clue how two hours had passed. I'd be surprised to find Annie B. at my feet waiting for her dinner; I didn't remember lunch.

I'd answer this question with a blank stare and, "I don't remember," or a long pause, then, "Little bit of this and little bit of that." This was the most truthful answer in the beginning months when my mind could neither focus nor finish anything.

Friends wanted more. "But how are you really doing, Tally?"

"Okay," I replied. Not fine, because I wasn't fine. But I was okay. I had okay hours and awful hours. Okay days and awful days. I never knew which awaited me. Did they want to hear about my pleas to the ceiling, "What do I do, Jack?" when everything, relied on me?

Kate, my therapist, regularly asked in those early years, "What are you feeling?"

The answer was often, "Cuisinart." Swirling. Mixed up. Emotions like a box of crayons tossed in a food processor, and, as the chips of color whipped by, I was asked to name just one. Nothing whole or clear. In a high school art class, I remembered mixing the primary colors together and creating brown. How did I feel? Brown.

The to-do list full of urgent paperwork and simple household chores fell onto the mental pile marked "Later" on days when I struggled to feed the dog and myself. Junk mail addressed to Jack accumulated in a shoebox. Such items only served to prove he once lived here. This isn't a dream; I'm not in "Pretend Lane," where I imagined that he would come home any minute.

Sometimes my hands felt too heavy to open a folder to see what was inside or to hold a pen to sign a document. I hid. I was too tired. Which folder demanded, *"This is very, very, very important and can't be ignored any longer?"* Where to begin? Even if I finished one day's tasks, there would be more tomorrow, so much more that I wouldn't see much progress. One step forward, two back. Why start? I sighed. I froze. I walked away. I crawled under the blanket.

Oh, yes, Annie B., I know, I know. It's time to get up and take care of you.

Lesson #3: All Chores Are Your Chores

After Jack died, all chores were mine and were all done to my standard of what "clean" was. I no longer ignored specks of food from flossing on the mirror, the shower stall with grimy corners, refrigerator shelves sticky from spills, or the tabletops' dusty surfaces where I wrote, "Dust me" inside a heart. Jack never saw those messages, nor did the chore. No more thinking to myself, "Let it go; it's good enough." He tried.

Locking up in the evening was one of Jack's jobs, now mine. In the evening, after taking Annie B out for her last walk, I began the close-the-house-down routine, beginning with locking the front door behind us. Across the ivory Berber carpet of the living room, I locked the slider and screen, then moved swiftly over the oak floor to lock the kitchen door. I went downstairs to make sure the garage door was closed. Lights out. I closed every window, except the high ones accessible only by a long ladder. Wouldn't Annie B or I hear the ladder being placed against the house, and the metal clank of someone climbing the rungs to those upper windows? How my mind created scary scenarios.

Hours later, my eyes popped open, and my heart raced. Did I lock that front door? I couldn't distinguish if the memory of turning the lock knob was earlier tonight or last night, or the night before that. Think, Brain, think! I growled at the empty side of the bed, "This is your job, Bubba, not mine."

I rose and grabbed my slippers at the foot of the bed, stirring Annie B. "Please don't ask to go out, Ms. B." In the summer moonlight entering from the large staircase window, I walked down the fourteen stairs, touched the lock, and returned to bed. The door was locked, and

I was wide awake. Angry. Not once, but several times over the year ahead, I rose to do the same task.

A newly purchased can of pepper spray sat inside my nightstand, and another in my purse. I even thought of purchasing a small handgun. Where did my self-confidence and self-reliance go? One day in the local grocery store parking lot, a store I had used for the last twenty years, I broke a fingernail on the door latch when I tried to open my car. When did I start locking the car in my own neighborhood in broad daylight? The burden of the entire house and my own personal safety weighed on my shoulders.

When Annie B wanted out at two in the morning, it was always "my turn." "Can you hold it, Ms. B? No? Are you sure? OK, let's go outside."

Lesson #4: The Widowed Brain Is Not a High-Functioning Brain

The widowed brain simply does not function well. If at all.

My mind became a sieve: simple mental math, names, items on a grocery list (often forgotten on the kitchen counter), details, deadlines, and awareness of time seeped out. Or my mind became frozen, like a computer program with no reset button or escape key. At the end of each week, one task was to collect my own scrawled notes from the back of envelopes, blank spaces on opened mail, napkins, the little pad in my purse, and another pad in the car. I once left a compiled list in the pocket of my shorts and washed my tasks and shopping list away in the laundry. I could not recall a single item on that piece of paper. Nothing.

I lived with apologies:

"I'm sorry, I forgot."

"I'm sorry, I don't remember."

"I'm sorry, I don't know."

I said those phrases so often that one would think I'd no longer be embarrassed. But I was. I stammered, cheeks flushed, ransacking my short-circuiting memory. I held my hands stiffly to my side or stuffed them in my pockets to keep myself from slapping the sides of my head. Think, Tally, think.

My house heard my anger when I yelled one of Jack's favorite words: "Fuck!" Those four letters held the rawness and dirty edge I needed. I shouted at the walls, "Fuck! No, no, no." I shook my fist at the ceiling and stomped on the floor. "I hate my fuckin' life. I hate it!" I wanted Jack back now.

My brain and behavior had become unfamiliar to me, and I wanted the old me back: the smart, mindful, cheerful, kind me. The happily married me.

Lesson #5: Holiday Traditions Cannot Stay the Same

It is like trying to dance a waltz to rock music: familiar steps forced into a different rhythm. Holidays are times when one wants desperately to return to what once was, times when I attempted to retreat to "Pretend Land," the land of denial. Sadly, every survivor must adjust or leave behind treasured traditions.

My second Thanksgiving without Jack, after a year of spending holiday meals at friends' houses, always returning to my own empty home and barren kitchen, I bought myself the smallest turkey available. I wanted the aroma in the house and leftovers for the weekend. I wanted to continue the tradition I'd observed since childhood. While shopping in the dessert aisle of the local Safeway, the sight of a wrapped half pumpkin pie stopped me cold, and my eyes teared up: there were others like me in need of a smaller portion. I paused to see if another single, kindred spirit picked one up. No one.

Appropriately, on Black Friday, a good color for my mood, I baked the turkey and made the dressing, Jack's favorite. I could see him in the kitchen chopping and sautéing celery and onion, tossing in the bread cubes, the scent of thyme and rosemary in the air, as he hummed with anticipation of the first bite. I wasn't a dressing lover like he was. But I made it in his honor.

At the dinner table, I swallowed only two bites of the dressing and later tossed the remaining contents of the large casserole dish down the disposal. This tradition needed to be changed. I detest wasting food, and I don't like dressing.

Lesson #6: All Answers Are Your Own

When the washing machine died just three months after Jack passed, I stood before the dead machine and remembered days when laundry was Jack's job, the days when I yelled at him, "What were you thinking?" as I pulled out a ruined silk blouse washed with jeans, a shrunken wool sweater dried with towels, or formerly white bras now pink. Without him, only I could ruin something in the wash. I missed his lack of housekeeping skills and his eagerness to learn how to do it right, if only to avoid being yelled at.

If Jack were still there, within a few hours, we would have carried the old washer up the seven stairs from the basement, heaved it into Jack's truck, dumped it at an appliance recycling lot, purchased a new one, and hooked it up. We would have a load running before dinner.

Can I do this alone? Could I figure out the sequential steps to remove the old and get a new one inside? I needed to know I had what it took to survive this minor glitch, a new challenge in being alone. Looking back, out of so many possible solutions, I saw that I took the cheapest, but not the easiest, option. Another person would have said, "Have you thought about…?" but I didn't ask anyone. After all those years of a second set of hands, ideas, opinions, and answers, now, when I asked, "*What do you think?*" I was on my own to answer.

What do you think? Those four words flittered off the walls of a well-lit mortgage office, seventeen months after Jack's death, when I bought my new house and arranged financing. The dark wood desks, walls with framed watercolor landscapes, and gray-blue industrial-grade carpet radiated a serious business atmosphere. The thirty-something woman in a smart gray suit pulled out forms needing signatures from the pile on her desk. Once signed, they were placed into a long legal-size manila folder, a copy for her and a copy for me. Most of the questions were simple, but I stumbled on one.

"Do you want a fifteen- or thirty-year mortgage?" she inquired.

Without hesitation, I turned to the chair on my left, but only got out, "What do you…" before I realized I was staring at an empty chair. My heart stopped mid-beat. "*Where is he?*"

I was alone making this major decision, one that would impact me, only me, for many years. My eyes welled up. Fear rose within. "*Oh, Bubba, whisper to me, help me. Which one?*" Silence. The kind woman waited for me to look up from the floor, wipe my nose and eyes, and answer, "The fifteen-year mortgage."

The washer took a full week to replace, but I did it. One down. What's next, God? I walked smugly out of the utility room.

When I relayed this story in a session, my therapist jumped upright in her chair and leaned toward me. "Don't ask. You'll get an answer."

Lesson #7: Every Meal Shows You the "New Normal"

In the first months after Jack's death, food prep for any recipe became too laborious, demanding step-by-step thinking. The pantry slowly emptied. Freezer and refrigerator shelves held little. After a month, neighbors and friends stopped bringing plastic containers of food. Their lives went on, and they thought mine did, too.

A fellow widow related that she ate jars of bacon bits for meals. "Hey, they're real bacon, not the artificial junk." The whole support group chuckled. Another widow found solace in a vodka bottle. One woman had no problem eating out alone, which saved shopping, prepping, and cleaning up. Personally, I ate nothing close to a balanced meal, sometimes drank too much red wine, and didn't care. Microwave popcorn was a staple for lunch and dinner, quick and thoughtless.

Jack's favorite caramels and chocolate-covered peanuts sat uneaten in small See's sampler boxes, purchased months before his passing. Who was I saving these for? My heart replied, *They are his candies.* An open jar of refried beans and a slab of cheese, Jack's favorite for quesadillas, molded. I felt ashamed for what I threw down the disposal when I knew every fifteen seconds a child dies in this world of hunger.

Large casserole dishes were replaced with smaller microwavable cookware for meals prepared from smaller cans, boxes, and bags. I had fewer leftovers.

"Your life has gotten smaller, too," every shrinking meal sang to me.

Like my German Irish mother, I drowned my steamed Brussels sprouts in vinegar, topped with ground pepper. This was the only food I liked that Mr. Will-Eat-Anything-Put-in-Front-of-Him Jack wouldn't touch.

"Ewww, sprouts tonight?" Jack would say as he entered the kitchen, his face scrunched like a disgruntled toddler as he watched me prep the vegetables. I usually waited until he was gone for an evening wrestling match or meeting to steam a bowl for myself.

Knowing he would never walk in the front door again, the first bite of the vegetable tasted bitter. I missed his squinted eyes and the turned-up nose, which were as much a part of the meal as the vinegar. Now, I enjoyed something he couldn't. Survivor's guilt threatened to ruin the dish. *Enjoy them,* I heard Jack's voice in my head. *Better you than me.* I remembered his grin and the sparkle in his eyes as I took another bite.

Lesson #8: Other Men Are Named Jack, Too.

Meeting someone also named Jack was startling the first time. Like, there should only be one man or boy ever to be called "Jack." That was plain silly thinking, but hearing his name in someone else's life unraveled me. A slap. When introduced to another Jack, the polite words of response, "Hello Jack," curdled on my tongue. I envied that other people were out there saying "Jack" every day, and someone answered. Their Jack had a place to eat and sleep. Their Jack was breathing. I wanted that.

The oven thermostat burned out. After baking some zucchini bread, I left the door open to let the heat out, but forgot to turn the oven off for several hours. Flipping through my phone for a repair service, only after an hour poring over the owner's manual to see if I could fix it myself, I saw a local repair business whose owner was named Jack. Oh, Jackson, are you pointing to this one? And laughing?

At the front door, I shook his hand and heard him say, "I'm Jack." No, you're not.

Having this Jack in my home was both comforting, I was in good hands again, and eerie.

Standing nearby as he worked, I heard my Jack say, "Get me that wrench," "Hold this end," or "Cut that two-by-four at sixteen and a half inches." I remembered leaving the room when my Jack's profanity took away the joy of working on a project together. Repairman Jack did not swear at all.

I was quiet with Repairman Jack. I stood nearby the range to watch, learn, and perhaps help, but was as useless as the dust found underneath the oven. He didn't need my assistance in pulling out the range or handing him tools. He left no scent of aftershave or sweat and needed only the signed check when he was finished.

"Thank you, Jack," I said as he left.

Lesson #9: "Not Yet" Is Okay.

For several months, Jack's most personal possessions remained in the exact spot he left them on the day he left this earth: his toothbrush and paste, razor and shaving cream, and comb on the bathroom counter; his books on the nightstand; beer in the garage mini-refrigerator; clothes in the closet and drawers. Even his favorite chair and spot on the couch couldn't be sat in by anyone, including me. As if he were coming back.

A year later, I sat in his rocking chair at the cabin. My eyes closed. I imagined his voice: It's time, Talle. It's OK to sit here. But I couldn't sit there comfortably. Eventually, I flipped the locations of our chairs, putting mine by the window where his rocker was. That rocker was still his. Sometimes I tossed my jacket or computer bag onto it, but if I sat there, it felt like I was sitting on his lap, crowding him. Not yet, Bud, I told him.

Lesson #10: The Hole in Your Heart Never Mends

I savor memories of Jack in a museum-like room in my heart, a gallery where I sit with him on a bench, admiring the large mosaic that hangs on one wall. Each colorful small chip is a piece of our conversations, ocean sunsets we saw, dogs we loved, our travels, birthday adventures, artwork we viewed and acquired, pillow-talk nights. All held by a frame of our twenty-six years of marriage. Such a masterpiece both soothes the pain of grief and reminds me of what once was. Smiles and sorrow. "Sweet bitter," not "bittersweet."

On the opposite wall is another mosaic, a portrait of widowhood: chips from a broken coffee mug and a wedding goblet, a replaced dryer, houses sold and bought, endless paperwork, my solo travels, and a new rescued dog. This piece honors my inner strength and courage, my willingness to admit that some things are out of my control.

When I need to sit with Jack, I open the blinds in this room, stir the dust, and watch the particles sparkle and float in the sunlight. I pick up his lime-scented aftershave from the shelf, open it, and inhale what smelled so good on him; see him in a suit before we left for an evening show; inhale it again with the lovemaking afterward. I brush off the framed picture of Jack wearing a PE teaching T-shirt and press it to my chest. My eyes fill while I speak to his blue-gray eyes. "I miss you so much. I love you."

Once, I surprised myself by saying, "I loved you." The past tense clanged. How did that happen? What corner of my mind had accepted the death and announced it aloud? I shook my head, holding that framed picture.

A widowed friend said, "The hole in your heart never mends." After letting that sink in, she continued, "But with time, the raw edges don't hurt as much."

Lesson #11: The Calendar Remembers, Too.

I recall the precise details of the afternoon medical appointment when Jack's melanoma diagnosis was given: the doctor's silvery hair, white medical coat, and her soothing, professional voice. The room's fluorescent lighting, the chrome table, and our plastic-backed chairs. That December 4th anniversary stood as a pillar marking the beginning of a path to his death on June 28, four years later. If I stop whatever I am doing and replay the memory, I am back in that office, or beside him on the bed the day he died, or on the ferry tossing his ashes into Puget Sound, like it was all this morning.

The calendar holds these events, too.

All the wedding anniversaries, birthdays (his and mine), Father's and Mother's Days, and winter holidays were difficult times. But unexpectedly, the week before Jack's death anniversary was worse than the day of. I was caught unaware that first year; I had anticipated the actual anniversary day would be the hammer, so I was surprised when I was pounded back into the earliest days of grief the week prior: I cried easily, sleep was elusive, and focus was impossible. I walked through the house searching for him, in the kitchen brewing his morning coffee, pulling his truck into the garage, the TV too quiet. Why was my life turned upside down again with such intensity? I punched pillows, stomped my feet, and yelled at God. I wore myself out so that the day of his death became anticlimactic.

Other widowed acquaintances related how they, too, found the days before an anniversary hellish.

I marked in purple ink on the dry-erase calendar "Jack's Anniv" on the 28th of every month for years, until the monthly anniversary became just another number on the calendar. One year, I simply noted aloud, "Jack passed today." The sorrowful pen dried.

Lesson #12: Time, That Four-Letter Word, Is the Healer.

Tears do slow from a torrent to a flow, and eventually a trickle, with the passage of time.

For months, I waited for that front door to open and Jack to stroll in wearing a new polo shirt embroidered with a conference logo and a wide grin, finally announcing, "I'm home." He had simply forgotten to tell me of an out-of-state meeting. We'd return to balance, routines, and comfort. Together. But when time uncurled my fists, how well I had held onto the sands of denial, nothing was left of the fantasy but a few fine grains caught between my fingers.

After Jack's death, I did what was once unfathomable, impossible: I lived alone for a whole year, followed by another. Slowly, my body and mind crawled out from "*This is my life without him*" toward "*This is my life.*"

In those first two years, I made the choice to live on, not to miss any once-in-a-lifetime experiences that came my way. Life was too precious. Fragile. Unpredictable. "Say yes to every invitation," another widow advised. Stamped into my passport is the ten-day East Mediterranean cruise I took alone, fifteen months after Jack's passing.

Another stamp shows ten days with a travel group in Egypt a year later. Seven months after returning from Egypt, I toured Ireland with a group, all widowed. And then Iceland, alone. I bought a house, painted the walls in new colors, filled it with new furniture, and found spots for the old. I planted bulbs for spring colors, my symbol that I survived the dark, cold winter. A new rescue dog sat on the passenger seat of my car and beside me on the couch. I missed Jack in every single second of those experiences, how much more fun they would have been with him by my side. But I did them.

I said, "Yes."

With time, I learned to trust myself with big decisions. If it were a big mistake, or if trying to fix it made things worse, I tried to be gentle with myself, although only after a good deal of swearing. "Be gentle," Kate advised, "trust yourself."

Lesson #13: Like a Train, Life Moves On, Whether You're on Board or Not.

I detest the phrase, "Oh, you have moved on," from those who know my story. Those words imply that I left my grief and love behind. Although I moved to a new house, I packed and brought the past with me. No, I have lived on. I made the hard choices to embrace what life I have left after Jack died. I carry our memories with me.

Widowhood was the most devastating experience of my six decades of life. Five years and hundreds of written pages later, I still do not have adequate words to illustrate the hell and torment I went through. I do my best with simple stories because nothing can accurately describe the experiences. Stories are exactly what bond the widowed to one another. We can simply ask, "How long did you hold onto his toothbrush?" and stories will spill from our hearts.

Hot molten steel is tempered by stretching it within seconds of its breaking point, at which point, when cooled, it is at its strongest. Widowhood was such a stretch. It threw me into the fires of apathy, anger, and confusion, and butted me up against *"Do I want to live?"* After passing this test, and I passed it, I am stronger and more sensitive to those who suffer loss. I am more than I ever imagined myself to be: stronger, more resolved, with greater perspective.

My pen stopped mid-air the first time an application asked for a check in a box:

☐ Married ☐ Single ☐ Divorced ☐ Widowed

For over twenty-six years, I marked the first box. I mark a new box, still missing the old one. Fate isn't always fair. Loved ones die too soon. Healing from grief doesn't have a neat formula with precise deadlines or established steps. "Moving on" is what life does, barreling forward year after year, whether we participate or not. Living on is a choice. It takes courage pulled from the very depths of your soul, and more strength than you thought possible. It is possible.

A smile does look back from the mirror eventually.

Chapter 31
Letter

My Dearest Jack,

I found a penny today, a very scratched-up one, on the sidewalk along my jogging route. After reading the year, I placed it in a pocket of my jacket. "Hi back at ya, Jackson," I said to the gray sky, hoping you were smiling back at me. I felt the penny in my pocket and wondered, *Were we together or apart in the year stamped on this penny? What were we doing if you were alive?* I do this with every penny I find.

I miss you so much. Those words gather in my chest and flitter about like frightened birds until I speak them. Words soothe the rustling of wings and soften my fears, but only for a moment. The fluttering always returns.

Sometimes it feels like you left only days ago, not five years. I still miss you with a force as strong as the raw grief of the early months, a grief that whisks me into a frenzy, sometimes a fury, at what my life became after your last breath. But those hard days have become fewer and farther apart with the years.

Who knew "alone" could be this lonely?

Talk to me, Jackson. Tell me about Heaven. Then I will share my ascent from Hell.

I should have written this letter to you sooner, to watch your hands unfold my words, a blush run from your collar to your ears, and moisture gather in those blue-gray eyes. I should have given you the chance to mumble your words of love back at me. But I didn't, nor did you.

Scrunched pages, attempts to write a perfect letter (yes, it must be perfect to speak of my love), are scattered around me. The words change with each day, deepened by a thunderstorm or moved by hearing one of our favorite songs playing over the store speakers in a grocery aisle. I have healed, learned, and evolved into someone new, day by day. I will write of yesterday's tears in today's words. Tomorrow's attempts at this letter will demand too *much* or not *enough,* and I will have to start over.

This task will never be finished if I don't let my inner perfectionist go. You know that part of me, don't you? We shared that trait. Remember our phrase when we realized we had pushed ourselves a bit too hard, to make remodeling jobs or school projects better and better, letting hours slip away on insignificant details?

"It's good enough," one of us would say to the other. So here is my best attempt today to tell of the last five years. My final attempt. *Good enough.* I'm smiling now, thinking those words, even though I know this isn't perfect.

I await those signs that you are near: the pennies, the dragonfly in the yard, or the feather that drops at my feet. I've found pennies in the street, in store aisles, even in the goalie box while playing soccer. The most stunning was the American penny I found while walking to the travel bus from the tourist shop in Ireland, pulling it out of a compressed dirt path. "Pennies from Heaven," I was told: our loved ones drop these reminders so we know they are watching us.

What were we doing in 1983, married only two years? Or in 2004, you had your first of several major surgeries to remove your lymph nodes. Later years, like 2009 on the copper: you'd been gone a full year, and I had moved from our house in Bellevue to my house in Kenmore. Pennies make me pause and remember.

You've become quieter; there are fewer heavenly messages.

The space between what was ours and what is now all mine has grown wider and longer with the passing years, stretching out like one of those long highways we drove to your parents' in Spokane, your birthplace, through the wheat fields of Eastern Washington, barely a curve or knoll, with a horizon that keeps on moving away. There are fewer reminders of you in my home; only the art we bought together and the memories that radiate from the walls and shelves.

The past and present are intertwined, woven. Twisted with our birthday adventures, barbecue dinners and huge salads, mocha mornings, and ice cream desserts, these are the things I remember. The things I do now are smaller and simpler: preparing smaller meals, avoiding our favorite café, and eating holiday dinners at friends' family tables.

On some days, your name still slips out as if you are in the other room. While reading the paper the other day, I said, "Jack, the Yankees are playing..." I paused, looked up, and finished softly to the empty chair, "...are playing Boston today." A piece of you, a piece of us, scooped out again from within my chest. The echoes return.

I attend the memorials of our former colleagues, cry for both of us, and ache for your hand to hold. This happens regularly, Jackson. Like stumbling on a small stone, I struggle to find my footing again, all because I wanted to share something I read, saw, or heard with you. Instead, I wrestle with reality: *He's not here.*

I miss you some days so excruciatingly that I must remind myself to inhale while sorrow blinds my eyes. I love… but I loved you? The past tense fits: *I was your wife, and we were married.* But *loved you?* I still stammer around verb tenses when you should be telling half the story with me.

During your last year of life, whenever I left the room, I kissed your lips or the top of your hairless head and said, "I will always love you." Every time. The words still ring true, even now.

You know that, don't you?

I miss mornings with you. Sitting at a table you never saw, I look out a kitchen window of a home with only my name on the contract, at the maple and cottonwood leaves I raked. I've watched five years of changing colors here. A glass mug of steaming Irish Breakfast tea, the color of stained walnut wood, awakens my morning energy. A new mug for the new house. And I think of you and our breakfasts at the old house. I can't make pancakes for one.

I think of the "DOG LOVER" mug, the survivor of the pair gifted by our neighbor Amy, the pair we used on so many weekend mornings in our house for our hot mochas. I thought it would be part of my days here. But I've used it only once. Without your mug, buried at the old house with its unexplained cracks, my mug seems out of place on the cabinet shelf, like a spring shirt hung among winter jackets. I can neither give it away nor use it.

The mug holds too much.

I also learned that I make a lousy mocha. On a snowy Sunday morning several months ago, I brought out the espresso machine we bought after retirement and tried to make your hot mocha. The paper was already spread on the table, waiting. Anna, a new rescue dog you would have loved, was nearby in her bed on the kitchen floor. (I fulfilled our dream of an old-dog rescue in our retirement years. I missed your affirmation, "Yeah, that's the one," when I chose a dog from the website.) Anna snoozed while I, in my typical comfy, weekend-worn sweats and a favorite Henley shirt, retrieved the mug, brewed the shot, frothed the soy milk, and squeezed in the chocolate syrup. Like so many of our rituals, I thought I could recreate this one and sip the warm memory while sitting at the table. But I failed: not hot enough, not enough chocolate, not enough foam. Had the coffee turned bitter? I poured it and my disappointment down the drain after only a few sips, and returned the cleaned mug to its shelf, never to try again.

After that, I watched dust gather on the espresso machine stored on the pantry floor. One day, I accepted a new truth: making mochas belonged with you at the old house, not here. I packed the thermometer, shot glass, frothing pitcher, and two demi-cups in a plastic grocery bag. Hugging the black-and-chrome device, "*Thanks for the memories,*" I handed the machine and bag to the attendant at a Goodwill drop-off. Back in the car, did you cry with me?

Your death has steeled and strengthened me as only a tragedy can. The word "Believe" is cut into a flat, fifteen-inch piece of copper and hangs in the bathroom here. I found it in a local art gallery just months after you left. A daily reminder. I cannot see my future, but I know something waits out there, it even peers into the windows of the house to see if I am ready, not as an intruder, but as a child waiting for her friend to come outside and play. I believe in tomorrows.

I must believe.

The hyacinths, gladiolas, tulips, daffodils, and whatever other bulbs I bought on impulse are poking green shoots from the well-mulched soil. I don't know which flower will bloom when or where;

only that when they do, I smile. They are last November's attempt to believe in a new life. The flowers represent survival, having made it through the Pacific Northwest's dark, wet winter, and a joyful shout into the spring light. A triumph.

But you knew I would survive and live on, didn't you, even when I doubted it myself?

No other experience has so deepened my understanding of who I am as placing your remains into the earth and then turning around to see only one shadow walk away. For a long time, the footing was slippery, backward, rarely gaining ground, or losing what I had just achieved. Until one day, seemingly unexpectedly, I realized I was standing at the top of a hill rather than in the bog. I could see the vista. You are my inspiration on this journey.

A friend once said that marriage is when you can't believe how mad you are at someone you love so much. You and I fought about what I thought were obligatory phone calls home when you were out late with the guys after a wrestling match, and the way you were a quick draw with the VISA card, though I gave only a cursory raised eyebrow when you pulled out the card for a dinner date. When paying the monthly bills, I wanted to see, "Amount owed: $0.00." My outrage ruined the first of most months and sent both of us into separate rooms until I cooled off. I have discovered that I, too, am quick to purchase what is not budgeted for. I swear at myself each month when the bill comes, and send an apology from my desk chair to you. We were a pair, weren't we?

With chemo brain, your frequent use of "I forgot," "You didn't tell me," or "That's not what you/the doc/the nurse/the technician said," drove me into furies. I battled to be an understanding caregiver, a good wife. I joked that I had scars on my tongue from biting back retorts.

Do you remember the final art piece we bought together? Two bronze characters, one at the base holding steady a steel cable that curls up fifteen inches to another character who has climbed to the top, aptly titled *At the End of the Rope,* although I added, "...Her Rope." Your eyes flicked at me when I renamed the piece, and I heard those eyes say, *"Was I really that bad?"* I said nothing and let the art speak, but it was that bad. I survived living with cancer and its impact on both of us, bodies and minds.

Now our monthly dry-erase wall calendar has been replaced by a smaller weekly magnetic version on the side of the refrigerator. I brought our calendar here, expecting to see the rainbow of pen colors on it again. I tried reassigning the colors: orange for the dog, blue for my friends, green for soccer, magenta for my therapist and doctor appointments. The red pen was yours, and for a few years, I wrote in your birthday. I used purple—a combination of my blue with your red—for the anniversaries of your death, until one day I forgot to mark the calendar.

The new kitchen is smaller, and there is no space above the phone to hang the monthly calendar. A smaller, simpler world without you. I live week to week. Your red pen denotes my soccer games and my writers' group. My blue pen covers everything from vet and medical appointments to meetings with friends, until both run dry. Green will become the next color to dominate the calendar, for no other reason than it's one of the oldest and will soon dry out, too. I miss our rainbow.

I haven't marked the monthly anniversary of your death for many months. Why? Because every day your memory hums from within me. Even when I think I have cleared out most of what was yours in the house, I find a love card tucked among the bills (which I re-tuck back), see your green bath towel at the cabin, or hear a song on the radio or my iPod, and I am flung back into your arms. The right song in the car brings you back as a passenger riding along with me, your Scottish, chiseled cheek-and-chin profile, a perfect, rugged lumberjack, off to the cabin, both of us dressed in flannel shirts and jeans. I hear you singing, as off-key as I.

When I am within the circle of people who loved you, your name easily slips into the conversation, as if I merely left you at home or in the car. With strangers, though, I hold your story tight inside. Too much needs to be said to explain what a great man and husband you were, to share how it all ended.

Whether I mark the calendar or not, my body knows: the week before the yearly anniversaries, the anniversary of your death, your birthday, and our wedding anniversary, a churn in my gut robs me of appetite, sleep, and clear thinking. The scars of grief are scratched at these times of year, and I bleed. I, the surviving spouse, hold the obligation to remember and honor those days. On May 9, I greet the morning with a silent, "*Happy Birthday, Jackson*," to the empty side of the bed. On June 28, the day of your passing, I start the day with, "*I miss you*," and I remind myself that I made it through another year without you. Dates are forever stored within me.

I am left with decisions, some easier than others: how and when to release my grip on our things, things that carry our stories. Of course, I kept Fergus, our traveling bear, and have packed him on several trips. Harder were your things. I passed many of your tools on to your son and that contractor friend of yours; they were too heavy for me to use safely. Needy men out there are wearing the clothes that used to belong in your closet and dresser drawers. Some got to shave or brush their teeth for a few weeks with your toiletries. Your meds helped a nurse in an AIDS clinic. Your death benefited many.

With "The Business of Death," your name came off all accounts we shared: credit cards, utilities, and even charity mailers. But regardless of how vigilant I was in contacting the sender of each "Mr. Jack Reynolds" piece of mail, every year an envelope addressed to you or "Mr. & Ms. Reynolds" arrives at this new house and steals my breath, yet brings a smile, a reminder that we were once a couple. Sadly, I make a note to update the sender.

The scab is scraped.

As your name and things left my physical world, I clutched the anger. You should not have died and left me to clean up alone. Were you given the peace you earned? I know you thought it was a sign of weakness that you did not beat the cancer. I know you suffered, but so did I. I need a target: someone responsible for the silence and for making me work so much harder to keep the house and cabin orderly. How the silence batters me. When there's nothing to grasp and shake and punch, I grab onto a moment and yell at the ceiling, "I need help, Jack. Now." I demand retribution from the damn cancer. Damn cancer for what it did to you. Damn cancer for what it did to me. The anger subsides slowly.

Whenever I retrieve my passport from the safe deposit box, I see yours. I pick it up from the red felt-lined box and open it. Unlike mine, yours doesn't hold any stamps, but your photo smiles up at me. I can't help but smile back as your eyes peer into mine. I miss the tickle of that mustache on my lips. Your face, those tortoise-rimmed glasses, your hair thinned on top, silver strands combed from a left-side part, are frozen at fifty-something, when we got the passport after our Mexico trip. Pre-cancer. My recent updated photo shows a loosening of skin around my eyes and neck, the crow's-feet deeper, and hair still brunette thanks to a good hair stylist. Aging is what happens while I fulfill our dreams. By the way, after all those travel classes we took on Greece, I made it there the year after you died. I hoped you stood behind me on the deck when the cruise ship headed to Athens, watched the full moon trail of light on the ocean, and held me tight for our twenty-seventh anniversary.

The caged birds are back within my chest, stirring about. I have to say the words again, Bud, because I cannot think until I set them free: I miss you. I miss you so much.

I imagine you in the vacant spaces next to me on planes, buses, taxis, and sidewalks. I miss you when I see a new barbecue spot or Italian restaurant, a road untraveled, a small-town event. I crave your "Let's go find out!" to my "What's over there?" Wandering aimlessly, among craft shows, local hardware stores, and county fairs, loses its spark of curiosity without you.

I do not know the day when my passport will join yours in the box. Until that day, I will embrace adventures and new smells, tastes, sounds, and sights. I want it said at my Celebration of Life that I lived to the fullest with the fewest regrets, not *I wished I had done that, but I chickened out.* Those are your final lessons, dear Teacher. It is cancer's lesson to survivors, too.

What is left of my heart to risk love again? "Through sickness and health" and "'til death do you part" are vows associated with real sorrows. One life will end sooner than the other. No longer innocent or naïve, I know what it costs to rebuild after a death, what it takes minute by minute. I learned how to live on, Jackson. But will I ever love with the depth we had? Will I hold back? I might hurt less if I love a little less. I don't know.

The safe deposit box also contains your wedding band, the band I had engraved with *Forever My Divine Love* thirty or so years ago.

Occasionally I pull out your ring from its box and hold it, notice the worn backside, and watch the small inset of diamonds flicker in the fluorescent light. Four years ago, my twin ring was resized, moved from my left to my right ring finger. Eventually, I took it off to rest in the narrow bank room of locked boxes, with yours.

The ring releases the memory of our wedding, holding your left hand in mine as I slide the ring on your finger. I see the light of the altar candles reflected in the ring, and the smile on your face as I recite my vows.

When I slide the safe deposit box into its metal slot, the bank teller locks the box in place and hands over my key. Your ring has the power to take me back to a time we believed we truly had eternity together. I am glad I didn't know how your life would end on the day I married you. Although if I did, I would have still married you. Here's the truth that stuns me: there is no forever, only a lifetime.

And yet, until we meet again, you will be forever my divine love. Tally

P.S. Give Annie B and Sneakers a hug for me whenever you play with them. See you all at the Rainbow Bridge someday.

ABOUT THE AUTHOR

Tally R. Reynolds is a retired educator who spent seventeen years as a teacher and fourteen years as a school counselor. In that career, she worked at nine different schools in the Seattle area. After experiencing widowhood, she felt compelled to write her memoir, believing newly widowed individuals might find comfort in recognizing both the similarities and differences in widows' stories.

She owns several "How to Write" books, all started but none finished. She lives in Kenmore, Washington, with her two small rescued chihuahua mixes. Life has continued to be full, playing soccer, working in her gardens, and always reading or listening to a book or two.

www.ingramcontent.com/pod-product-compliance
Lightning Source LLC
Chambersburg PA
CBHW051544030726
47592CB00001B/120